Keeping Your Child Healthy in a Germ-Filled World

A JOHNS HOPKINS PRESS HEALTH BOOK

Keeping Your Child Healthy in a Germ-Filled World

A GUIDE *for* PARENTS

Athena P. Kourtis, M.D., Ph.D., M.P.H.

THE JOHNS HOPKINS UNIVERSITY PRESS

Baltimore

Note to the reader: This book describes how to help prevent infections in children *in general*. It was not written about *your* child. You should obtain the services of a competent professional whenever you need medical or other specific advice.

Dr. Kourtis's work was performed outside the scope of her employment as a U.S. government employee. Her work represents her personal and professional views and not necessarily those of the U.S. Centers for Disease Control and Prevention.

The Johns Hopkins University Press
2715 North Charles Street
Baltimore, Maryland 21218-4363
www.press.jhu.edu

Library of Congress Cataloging-in-Publication Data
Kourtis, Athena P.
    Keeping your child healthy in a germ-filled world : a guide for parents / Athena P. Kourtis.
        p.   cm. (A Johns Hopkins Press health book)
    Includes bibliographical references and index.
    ISBN-13: 978-1-4214-0211-6 (hardcover : alk. paper)
    ISBN-13: 978-1-4214-0212-3 (pbk. : alk. paper)
    ISBN-10: 1-4214-0211-4 (hardcover : alk. paper)
    ISBN-10: 1-4214-0212-2 (pbk. : alk. paper)
    1. Self-care, Health—Popular works. 2. Microorganisms—Popular works. I. Title.
    RA776.95.K68 2011
    613—dc22   2011004100

A catalog record for this book is available from the British Library.

Illustrations by Elizabeth Allen

Special discounts are available for bulk purchases of this book. For more information, please contact Special Sales at 410-516-6936 or specialsales@press.jhu.edu.

The Johns Hopkins University Press uses environmentally friendly book materials, including recycled text paper that is composed of at least 30 percent post-consumer waste, whenever possible.

To Alexander,
and to Peter and Constantine,
the three "Greats" in my life!

"The physician must ... have two special objects in view
with regard to disease, namely, to do good or to do no harm."
—Hippocrates, *Epidemics,* fifth century BC

Contents

PART II

Our Defenses against Germs

Preface

When you hold this book in your hands, the last thing on your mind, I am sure, is the number of germs moving from your hands to its surface. Germs are microscopic organisms present everywhere: in the air, on the ground, in water, on plants and animals, in the human body. They live in tropical and polar climates, near volcanoes and hot springs, with or without oxygen.

Since the nineteenth century, we have known that some germs cause diseases—the infectious diseases. Around the end of the twentieth century, however, scientists began to understand that germs also cause chronic diseases, such as stomach ulcers and some types of cancer. New scientific evidence has started to connect germs with even more diseases, including atherosclerosis, diabetes, some forms of arthritis, and neuropsychiatric conditions. However, not all germs are enemies. Even though some germs cause disease in humans, animals, and plants, many of them are necessary for our health. In fact, we would not be able to exist without them.

The relationship between humans and germs is complex and fragile. They can damage our health—even kill us—but we need them for our very existence. Since we cannot eliminate all germs (and we do not want to), how can we live healthily *with* them? What should we do to protect ourselves and our children from germs, without endangering our health from the harmful consequences of our protective measures? Should we clean our homes? Should we vaccinate our children? Should we use antibiotics? How about antibacterial soaps? Information piles up as the media and the Internet step in to offer (sometimes conflicting) advice.

Inspired by the questions of my little patients' parents, I wrote this book to help you sift through the media information you receive daily. As a *pediatrician*, I have the privilege of serving my patients—children and their families—and I hear the questions and see the worries parents have about their children's health. However, I also see the extent of misinformation that is circulated: some parents believe that antibiotics are a cure-all, other parents have misgivings about vaccines, and still others fall prey to the wide promotion of products and ideas with no scientific backing. As an *infectious diseases specialist*, I see some of the more serious cases of infectious diseases in children, as well as nosocomial infections (those acquired in the hospital) and infections caused by germs that are resistant to antibiotics. As a *mother*, I know firsthand what concerns parents and what information they truly need to know.

It is my mission to help educate parents on infections and their prevention as related to their children's health. I begin with an introduction to germs to give you some background about them and their ongoing relationship with humans. The first part of this book describes what germs your children are likely to encounter through their various activities. I describe how these germs spread and multiply and how they make us sick. Understanding how germs spread and the pathways they use is the first step to preventing infections.

The second part of this book discusses the means we have today for preventing infections: new ways of practicing hygiene for ourselves and for our home, whether we should use antimicrobial soaps and cleaning products, and the very important preventive strategy offered by vaccines. Part II also explores the proper use of antibiotics, prevention of infections during pregnancy, the benefits of breastfeeding, and whether our children's immune systems require food supplements or herbs. Probiotics is a new and evolving field; I describe what we know about these live microorganisms that some people take to improve their health. Finally, I talk about traditional wisdom and folk remedies and whether they have any scientific merit in preventing and treating infectious diseases.

You can read this book from beginning to end or use it as a reference for specific questions that you have. I hope that it will be helpful for a new generation of parents and that it will set the foundation for carefully evaluating the information we receive and carefully handling the situations we encounter every day. By applying what you learn from this book, you can reduce the frequency of infections in your family and better understand our fragile ecological balance with microbes.

Acknowledgments

As the poet George Seferis said, "Our words are children of many people."
This book would not have been possible without the help of many people
during the course of my studies and work. The idea for this book started
from a conversation with my mother, but its foundation was laid much earlier. I owe gratitude to my parents, who encouraged me along the path of
knowledge and creation; my teachers all the way from elementary school to
medical school and throughout my medical and research training, who introduced me to "brave new worlds"; my colleagues, with whom I continue to
share knowledge; and my patients and their families, who continually offer
me new challenges.

To my husband and sons, who were patient and forgiving of my absences
for hours—day and night—as I spent my free time writing, I extend my heart-
felt thanks. My special thanks to my father, Dr. Petros Kourtis, a general
surgeon, to my husband, Dr. Alexander Kessler, an infectious diseases specialist, and my colleague Dr. Andi Shane, a pediatric infectious diseases
specialist, who read various parts or all of my manuscript and provided
thoughtful and useful comments. Jacqueline Wehmueller, executive editor
at the Johns Hopkins University Press, believed in this project from the
beginning, and Rowena Rae, my enthusiastic editor, made the book much
more interesting to read. Finally, to my publishing team, which made the
process, despite the hard work, exciting, I express my deep gratitude.

Keeping Your Child Healthy
in a Germ-Filled World

When Germs and People Interact

AN INTRODUCTION

Germs, also called microorganisms or microbes, have been on Earth for more than three and a half billion years, making them the oldest living organisms. They are generally classified in four groups:

1. Bacteria are single-cell organisms that are just a few thousandths of a millimeter in size.
2. Viruses are infectious agents—technically not even organisms, because they can only multiply within other organisms—and are much smaller than bacteria.
3. Fungi are a type of plant and include microscopic yeasts and molds.
4. Parasites are organisms that live in or on a host organism and include microscopic single-cell protozoa and larger, nonmicroscopic parasites such as the helminths (worms).

Germs that cause diseases are labeled pathogenic. In reality, though, less than 1 percent of all germs cause disease in humans. About 100 billion bacteria live on our skin, and another 100 billion in our mouth. Our intestinal tract is covered by almost 100 trillion bacteria. Far from making us ill, these bacteria are beneficial to us. For example, many bacteria, such as some species of *Lactobacillus*, live in our intestines and help us to digest food, destroy pathogenic bacteria, fight against cancer cells, and produce necessary vitamins. The body's immune system helps us to survive in the sea of microbes by learning, in infancy, to differentiate harmless and harmful bacteria. Thus, our immune system recognizes

1

that the former are to be tolerated and the latter attacked, and, most of the time, the immune system does so quickly and effectively.

Germs and Humans throughout History

Although so few germs cause diseases, the pathogenic (disease-causing) germs, not surprisingly, are the ones we hear about most frequently. Pathogenic germs have caused infectious diseases in humans for millennia, possibly since the time of the first civilizations. Evidence of infections has been found in prehistoric humans, who may even have used natural remedies against them. For example, in the intestine of the Iceman, a frozen mummy found on the mountains of northern Italy and believed to have lived between 3300 and 3100 BC, scientists found the eggs of a parasite, *Trichuris*. They also discovered among the Iceman's possessions the fruit of a birch fungus, which contains substances toxic to intestinal parasites. Perhaps prehistoric humans had identified this fungus as antiparasitic and were using it as a remedy.

There is no question that infectious diseases have played a central role in human history. Smallpox, described in ancient Egyptian and Chinese texts, is an infectious disease that has had a particularly large impact. Many researchers believe that over the centuries smallpox has caused more deaths than all other infectious diseases combined. The disease was eradicated from the world through a massive and coordinated immunization program against the smallpox virus; the last case occurred in 1977. To date, smallpox is the only human infectious disease that has been eliminated.

Malaria, mentioned in Egyptian texts and described in detail by Hippocrates, has also had a huge impact. Transmitted through the bite of mosquitoes that carry a parasite called *Plasmodium*, malaria was a scourge during the Roman Empire. Today, many swamps, where mosquitoes breed, have been drained, so malaria seldom occurs in Europe and North America. However, it continues to kill millions of people in the world's tropical regions, and given the climate changes anticipated for the future, malaria is likely to expand into areas that today are not considered tropical, just as West Nile virus infection and dengue fever have.

Bubonic plague, another dreaded infectious disease, was spread in Europe, Africa, and the Middle East by fleas carried on rodents that arrived in merchant caravans from Mongolia. In the fourteenth century, bubonic plague killed 20 million people in Europe alone, earning it the label "black death." Plague is caused by a bacterium transmitted to humans from a fleabite; the fleas become infected when they bite infected rodents, such as rats. Today, this disease is rare, but it does still occur.

Tuberculosis, caused by a mycobacterium and spread through the air, is an ancient disease that has plagued humans throughout history; indeed, evidence of it has been found in prehistoric skeletons and in Egyptian mummies dating from the fourth millennium BC. Romanticized in the eighteenth and nineteenth centuries and linked to artistic talent and temperament, tuberculosis nevertheless caused millions of deaths until antibiotics were discovered in the mid-twentieth century and higher standards of hygiene, nutrition, and living conditions emerged. Tuberculosis remains the leading cause of death worldwide from a curable infectious disease, and the new mycobacterial strains are more dangerous because they have become resistant to many antibiotics.

Influenza, or the flu, is another example of an infectious disease with a large impact on human history. Widespread epidemics, called *pandemics*, of flu have occurred several times during the twentieth century. The most severe flu pandemic, in 1918–19, caused between 20 million and 40 million deaths worldwide. There have been more flu pandemics over the intervening years, and we recently went through another one, the H1N1 pandemic, which was not as severe as others have been.

The human immunodeficiency virus (HIV), which leads to AIDS, has caused a new pandemic. In 2008 alone, HIV/AIDS killed about 2 million people worldwide, and another 33 million were living with the virus.

People's Perceptions: How We Think about Germs

In the 1960s and 1970s, many scientists believed that modern medicine had "defeated" infectious diseases. In the two previous decades, the 1940s and 1950s, scientists discovered antibiotics and produced many new vaccines. This golden era of antibiotics and virology coincided with the development of insecticides and with tremendous progress in food preservation technologies. All these advances meant that many infectious diseases, which had previously threatened human health, appeared to have been defeated or controlled. In addition, with refrigeration widely used and modern methods in place for food production and processing, many people thought that hygiene was obsolete and redundant, and they stopped teaching their children about basic hygiene practices.

Humankind seemed to be less vulnerable to infections than ever before. In 1962, the microbiologist McFarlane Burnet, a Nobel laureate, prefaced a new edition of his book *Natural History of Infectious Disease* with "at times one feels that to write about infectious diseases is almost to write of something that has passed into history." Today, with the benefit of hindsight, this statement appears complacent and arrogant. Indeed, in the past few years, scientists have come to recognize two different phenomena, both of which have radically changed the way we perceive germs.

The first phenomenon is the appearance of new germs and the reappearance of old ones that were on the verge of disappearing. The new germs include the avian flu and swine flu viruses, the severe acute respiratory syndrome (SARS) virus, the West Nile virus, the parasite *Cryptosporidium*, the bacterium *Legionella*, and, of course, HIV, the AIDS virus. About thirty new pathogenic germs have appeared in the last thirty years! Infectious diseases that have reappeared after having been controlled include poliomyelitis, tuberculosis, malaria, and a series of infections caused by germs that have developed resistance to antibiotics, an example of which is methicillin-resistant *Staphylococcus aureus* (MRSA).

We should not be surprised, because the genetic makeup of germs, like all living organisms, continually evolves as germs multiply. Thus, germs are able to infect other animal species, become less susceptible to antibiotics, and alter their response to a host's immune defenses. Lately, these changes are occurring much more frequently. The worrisome acceleration in the rate at which germs are evolving results from a combination of factors, all related to human changes. We have adopted new behaviors, new methods of food production and processing, and new modes of rapid transportation, all of which promote the transmission and spread of germs. Advances in medical treatments and some new diseases have led to longer survival of patients with weakened immune defenses and greater vulnerability to infections.

Both the human population and the ease of global travel have increased greatly, leading to humans encroaching on more and more of the planet. Urbanization, industrialization, and changes in farming and animal husbandry have led to humankind destroying some ecosystems and altering the ecologic relationships of many others. As a result, pressure is put on germs, and this pressure causes them to evolve. Even medical and public health practices have pushed germs to evolve. A prime example is the overuse of antibiotics, which has contributed to a great problem in medicine today—difficult-to-treat infectious diseases caused by germs that have become resistant to antibiotics.

Other human-induced factors are also significant. Increases in both the exotic animal trade and forest destruction have led to greater opportunities for animal germs to jump to humans. From time to time, when the combination of pressures is just right, a previously harmless germ can evolve into one that is pathogenic for humans, as likely happened with the viruses that cause AIDS, SARS, and avian flu. Wars, natural disasters, and economic and political upheaval all affect the status of germs and infectious diseases. For example, economic and political changes in the early 1990s that brought about the collapse of public health systems in eastern Europe allowed dangerous diseases that had been quelled, like diphtheria, to resurface.

The World Health Organization (WHO) estimated that in 2004 alone, infectious diseases were responsible for over 10 million deaths worldwide, making infections the primary cause of fatalities in the world. While the number of deaths from infectious diseases has decreased in developed countries, the total number of infections has not changed. What have changed are the *types* of infections. For example, cholera and typhoid fever were prominent one hundred years ago, whereas today, there are more viral infections and recently emerged infections, like those caused by the bacteria *Campylobacter* and *Legionella*, the parasite *Cryptosporidium*, and HIV. The developing world still struggles with bacterial, viral, parasitic, and fungal infections that have become less common in developed countries but that continue to take the lives of millions of children and adults every year.

The second phenomenon that has become apparent recently is the large increase in the frequency of allergic conditions (asthma and other allergies) and autoimmune diseases (such as lupus, some types of arthritis, type 1 diabetes, and ulcerative colitis). The reasons behind these increases are not well understood, but some scientists have suggested that extreme cleanliness and antibiotic overuse (both in people and in animals) may be responsible.

A theory called the *hygiene hypothesis* proposes that our immune systems need a certain level of germs in the environment to be "educated" not to overreact to environmental stimuli. The proponents of this theory claim that a lack of germs, because of either a high level of hygiene or the excessive use of antibiotics and vaccinations, may have caused immune systems to become misguided and confused, resulting in the appearance of more allergies and autoimmune disorders in Western societies. In other words, the war that we declared against germs may have caused collateral damage to humans.

Many people simplified the hygiene hypothesis and declared that antibiotics, vaccines, and "excessive" cleanliness are enemies. Books and newspaper articles proliferated with titles like "Let Your Children Be Dirty." I discuss the hygiene hypothesis in detail in Part II of this book, but suffice it here to say that harmful results of misinformation have already appeared. In the United States and in some European countries, more and more parents have stopped vaccinating their children. As a result, diseases that had almost disappeared, such as measles, pertussis (whooping cough), and mumps, have now staged a comeback.

Thus, these two phenomena make it clear that we cannot disregard germs; we still have much to learn about them and their interactions with humans. What does the future hold? We cannot (and we would not want to) destroy all germs, but we can lessen the harmful consequences of some that cause infections, while maximizing the benefits that our coexistence with others offers to our health and our children's health. As parents, we have the essential role of protecting our children in a safe yet sensible way and of teaching them how to protect themselves as they navigate their lives through the microbial world.

PART I

Which Germs Where?

1

I'm Hungry!

FOOD-BORNE GERMS AND
FOOD PREPARATION SAFETY

As parents, we are naturally concerned about the quality of food our children eat. Food provides the necessary energy and nutrients for children to survive and grow, but food can also harbor germs that make people ill. No parent would knowingly give a child contaminated food, yet food poisoning occurs in children, and adults, all too frequently. Most of the time, these food poisoning incidents are entirely preventable by following a few rules about food storage and preparation, as well as being aware of the risks associated with certain foods and locales.

In this chapter, I focus on the microorganisms that can be found in food and the risks these microbes pose to children. You will find a "quick look" at food-borne illness in table 1.1. I do not discuss the effects of preservatives, additives, or potentially toxic substances like pesticides or fertilizers that may be found in foods, nor do I discuss food allergies. In a later chapter, however, I describe the role of diet in the development of a child's immune system, and I explore whether there is scientific truth in promoting certain substances as ingredients that strengthen the immune system.

What Are Food-Borne Germs and
Where Do They Come From?

Typically, germs are microorganisms, or microbes, and include bacteria, viruses, parasites, and fungi. As I discussed in the book's introduction, most germs are not harmful to humans. Some germs, however—called pathogenic germs, or *pathogens*—cause disease. A food-borne germ, therefore, is a pathogenic bacterium, parasite, or virus that is transmitted in food and causes illness in a person who eats the food. A person can also become ill from ingesting toxins, which are chemical substances produced by bacteria. Some bacteria in food will not cause illness themselves, but their toxins do. I use the general term *food poisoning* to identify a food-borne illness, regardless of whether the cause is a germ or a toxin.

The most common cause of food poisoning is a bacterium called *Staphylococcus*, often shortened to staph. Staph bacteria are found on many people's skin and hands and may cause skin infections such as boils, cellulitis, or abscesses. If someone who handles food is a staph bacteria carrier, the bacteria or their toxins can get on the food being prepared. Most staph food poisonings occur with foods high in protein, such as cooked meat, poultry, and fish, dairy products, mayonnaise, potato salad, and cream-based desserts. The symptoms of staph food poisoning start within only a few hours of consuming the contaminated food. The affected person will have symptoms of nausea, vomiting, and abdominal pain, which usually resolve in a few hours (three to four hours in babies; six to eight hours in older children and adults).

Several other germs frequently cause food-borne illnesses:

- *Salmonella* bacteria are usually thought of in connection with foods like raw meat, raw or undercooked eggs, and unpasteurized milk, but they can also be found on fruits and vegetables. Thorough cooking destroys *Salmonella*. The bacteria can be transmitted to people from animals as well, particularly from turtles and other reptiles (see chapter 4).
- *Clostridium perfringens* is a soil bacterium that can contaminate food from the unclean hands of a person preparing the food. It usually multiplies in canteens or buffets, where foods like beef, poultry, fish, stews, casseroles, and other cooked foods remain at room temperature for several hours.
- *Clostridium botulinum* is a bacterium that does not like oxygen, so it typically multiplies in canned food. Under certain conditions, its spores produce a dangerous toxin called *botulinum toxin*, which

causes muscle paralysis. The resulting illness is called botulism. (This is the same toxin used in Botox injections.)

Many other germs can also cause disease if an infected person contaminates food or water. Examples are the bacteria *Campylobacter* and *E. coli*, the hepatitis A virus, noroviruses, and parasites like *Cryptosporidium*. Table 1.1 lists the main germs and toxins that cause food poisoning, which foods each one is most commonly associated with, and some helpful information about each one. Note that of all food-borne illnesses, only one—hepatitis A—can be prevented with a vaccine. I discuss this vaccine more in chapters 6 and 9.

Many food-borne germs cause similar symptoms: nausea, vomiting, abdominal pain, diarrhea, and sometimes fever or jaundice (yellow color of the skin and eyes). Some types of food poisoning are particularly dangerous; for example, botulism can cause death by paralyzing the muscles that allow a person to breathe. How quickly symptoms occur depends on which germ or toxin is responsible. Symptoms of food poisoning can develop as quickly as a few hours after consuming contaminated food, as in the case of infection by toxin-producing staph bacteria, and as long as three to four days later, as in some cases of *Salmonella* or *Shigella* infection.

In terms of its microbial content, our food is much safer today than it was two or three generations ago, due to refrigeration and progress in animal husbandry and meat processing, among other scientific and technological achievements. Also immensely helpful has been the wide application of public health regulations, such as those for healthy transport and handling of animals in abattoirs and those for prewashing of packaged fresh vegetables. Despite these advances, however, diseases caused by food continue to occur, even in developed countries, and much more frequently in the world's poorer countries—the destination of more and more people who travel for recreation. According to estimates by the Centers for Disease Control and Prevention (CDC), food-borne pathogens cause illness in 75 million people every year in the United States. Of these people, 325,000 are hospitalized, and 5,000 die.

There are several reasons so many people become ill every year from food-borne germs. In many instances, poor hygiene by people preparing

TABLE 1.1
The most common food-borne illnesses, including causes, usual food sources, risk factors, and related information

Germ or toxin	Usual food sources	Risk factors	Season of greatest risk	Additional information
Bacterial toxins from *Staphylococcus*	Ham, poultry, cream-based desserts, potato salad, mayonnaise	Inadequate refrigeration (temperature over 50°F)	Summer	
from *Bacillus cereus*				
• Vomiting syndrome	Fried rice	Inadequate reheating of cooked rice (to less than 140°F or steaming hot)	Year-round	
• Diarrheal syndrome	Beef, pork, poultry	Advance preparation and inadequate refrigeration of cooked food (temperatures between 50°F and 140°F)	Year-round	
from *Clostridium botulinum*	Home-canned and jarred foods, commercially canned meats, honey	• Improper storage or preservation of home-canned and jarred foods • Risk from honey only in babies	Year-round	• Causes gastrointestinal (GI) symptoms and muscle paralysis • In a baby, causes constipation, weak cry, decreased appetite, paralysis
from *Clostridium perfringens*	Beef, poultry, gravy	Inadequate refrigeration of cooked food (temperatures between 50°F and 140°F)	Fall, winter, spring	

Bacteria				
Campylobacter	Poultry, certified raw or unpasteurized milk	Mainly in young people	Summer	
E. coli	Beef (especially ground beef); unpasteurized milk, cider, and juice; lettuce; seed sprouts; vegetables grown in fields where cattle have grazed	Transmission from a sick person to other people is common (called secondary transmission)	Summer, fall	A particular type of E. coli, labeled O157:H7, can cause toxin production and kidney failure in children (hemolytic uremic syndrome)
Listeria	Soft cheeses, unpasteurized milk, undercooked meat, deli meats (ham, salami, etc.)	High risk in pregnant women, newborn infants, and patients with AIDS, cancer, diabetes, kidney insufficiency	Summer	
Salmonella	Beef, poultry, pork, eggs, dairy, fruits, vegetables, seed sprouts, well water	Inadequate cooking	Summer	
Shigella	Mayonnaise, lettuce	Secondary transmission is common	Summer	
Vibrio species	Seafood, especially raw oysters	Raw seafood	Summer, fall	Most common in Gulf Coast areas
Yersinia	Pork, chitterlings, tofu, unpasteurized milk	Increased risk in patients with thalassemia (a red blood cell disorder)	Winter	

(continued)

TABLE 1.1 *Continued*

Germ or toxin	Usual food sources	Risk factors	Season of greatest risk	Additional information
Viruses				
Hepatitis A virus	Seafood, fruits, lettuce, sandwiches, any food handled by an infected person who doesn't use proper hygiene		Year-round	A vaccine is available
Norovirus	Seafood, salads, rice, water, ice		Year-round	
Parasites				
Cyclospora and *Cryptosporidium*	Raspberries, lettuce, tomatoes		Summer	

Other agents

Agent	Food	Source	Season	Symptoms
Fish toxins, including histamine (scombroid), ciguatera, and other neurotoxins	Tuna, mahimahi, bonito, mackerel, mussels, shellfish	• Inadequate refrigeration of uncooked fish (temperatures between 50°F and 140°F) • Shellfish harvested in areas with a red tide	Year-round	Causes neurological symptoms: headache, nausea, skin numbness or tingling (paresthesias), paralysis
Mushroom toxins			Spring, fall	Can cause severe gastroenteritis, liver and kidney failure, neuropsychiatric symptoms, hallucinations, coma, death
Heavy metals (copper, cadmium, zinc)	Lemonade, soft drinks, punch	Drinks in corroded metal containers		
Monosodium glutamate (MSG; added to improve flavor)		Chinese restaurants, fast food restaurants, and prepared food manufacturers often use MSG	Year-round	Causes paresthesias, headache, nausea, abdominal pain

and cooking food is to blame. In other cases, food is stored or cooked incorrectly. In addition, more and more foods, especially fruits and vegetables, are imported from around the world. Although food importation gives us the opportunity to eat exotic foods and foods that are not in season locally, it also multiplies the opportunities for germ transmission.

For example, in 1997, there were outbreaks of hepatitis A caused by frozen strawberries from Mexico; the strawberries are believed to have been tainted by irrigation water contaminated with human feces. In 1998, outbreaks of *Cyclospora*—a parasite that causes diarrhea and abdominal pain—were due to contaminated raspberries that had been imported from Guatemala. Diarrheal outbreaks from *E. coli* bacteria occurred in 2006 when people ate at a well-known fast food restaurant where hamburgers made with contaminated beef had not been cooked well enough.

Recently, *E. coli* bacteria have contaminated unpasteurized apple juice and packaged fresh spinach. Both products were available in supermarket chains and caused many people to become ill with diarrhea, and a few people to die. It turned out that the apples used to make the juice had fallen on ground soiled with cow feces—the *E. coli* bacteria are normally found in the intestinal tract of humans and animals—and the apples had not been adequately washed before squeezing. A similar scenario happened with the spinach.

Medical "detectives" at the CDC investigate outbreaks of food-borne illness by accumulating information about the time, place, and people infected and by making inferences about the origin of the germ, the food responsible for transmitting the germ, and the way in which the food became contaminated. Doctors use various tools, including epidemiology studies that examine the health and illness of populations of people, microbiological analyses, and molecular methods that shed light on the genetic origin of a germ (similar to a paternity test). Typically, when at least two people who ate the same food develop symptoms of a gastrointestinal illness (such as vomiting, diarrhea, abdominal pain, or fever), it is considered to be an outbreak of a food-borne disease.

Infants and children are more vulnerable than adults to the harmful effects of food poisoning, because their immune systems are much less experienced. In addition, children often suffer more than adults when they contract a food-borne illness. Children's smaller size makes it much easier for them to become dehydrated from losing fluids through vomiting and diarrhea. Food poisoning caused by the toxins of some bacteria, such as *E. coli,* can cause serious health problems in a child, including kidney failure and the breakage of red blood cells (hemolytic uremic syndrome, HUS); this syndrome sometimes leads to a child's death.

What is the best way to protect children from food-borne diseases? Two things are key: (1) being constantly aware of the potential presence of germs, and (2) establishing good basic hygiene habits. When we become parents, many of us change some of our everyday practices to ensure that the youngest and most vulnerable member of our family lives and grows in as healthful an environment as possible. I believe that having a child provides an excellent opportunity to relearn good habits for food preparation and consumption at home and when visiting restaurants and food markets, as well as the opportunity to teach these habits to our children.

A Home-Cooked Meal: Food Safety in the Kitchen

Following certain procedures in the home kitchen will go far in preventing food-borne illness from home cooking. One in five cases of food-borne illness, and nearly every *Salmonella* food poisoning, occurs from food prepared at home. When one member of a household has been infected with *Salmonella*, about 60 percent (or two of every three) of the other household members will also become sick, mainly by sharing a contaminated toilet.

What is the single most important thing you can do to minimize the chances of food poisoning? You have undoubtedly heard it many times before: Wash your hands! Wash your hands well with soap and water before you start preparing food, and wash them again while you are preparing food, especially when you have handled raw meat, poultry, or eggs. Insist that your children wash their hands before they eat and before they help you in the kitchen. Make hand washing a ritual with children and it will become a lifelong habit that will serve them well. And, of course, always wash your and your children's hands after using the toilet—a basic rule that some people overlook when they are in a hurry. I discuss hand washing in more detail, including different types of soap, in chapter 13.

In addition to the simple and effective wash-your-hands rule, there are several practices to keep in mind as you prepare, cook, and store food and as you clean up the kitchen afterward.

Food Preparation

Germs are commonly found on raw produce, particularly on meats, but also on vegetables and fruits. Rinse salads and fruits well with water—change the water at least twice—even if the package indicates that they are prewashed. With vegetables like lettuce and cabbage, remove the exterior leaves, which have the highest chance of being contaminated with germs or pesticides. Always prepare raw vegetables and fruits on a separate surface from the one you used to cut raw meats, and wash knives and other utensils when switching from raw meats to vegetables and fruits.

Working with raw meat, poultry, and fish requires a little more care and attention, because they harbor germs (like *E. coli, Salmonella, Campylobacter,* and others). If you place raw meat products on the kitchen counter or in the sink, clean these surfaces afterward with warm water and soap, followed by a light solution of bleach (one tablespoon of bleach in about one quart of water). Also wash the meat-cutting surface with water and soap followed by a bleach solution. Plastic surfaces may be more appropriate than wood because they are easier to clean, and if you have a dishwasher, the plastic surface can go directly into the machine for better cleaning. Recent studies in the United States and France showed that households using only soap and water or only wiping surfaces after preparing raw meat or poultry had about a threefold greater risk of gastrointestinal infections compared with households that cleaned surfaces in the dishwasher or with bleach. Knives and other utensils, as well as plates and serving dishes used for raw meat, must also be washed before they are used again.

Frozen meat or poultry should not be thawed overnight on the kitchen counter. The safest place to thaw frozen items is in the refrigerator, which means you need to allow a little more time for defrosting. Also, meats should be marinated in the refrigerator, not on the kitchen counter. Never reuse a marinade, because it has been contaminated with raw meat juices.

Try to think of the possible pathways for germs to get from one place

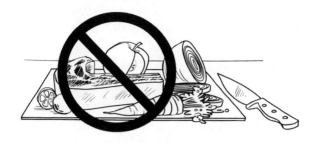

to another, and then do what you can to eliminate the pathway. For example, you might cut raw meat and then turn on the kitchen faucet. If there were any germs on the meat, they got onto your hands, and they are now on the faucet, which your child might later turn on to get a glass of water to drink while she eats her sandwich. Or you might use a towel to wipe up raw meat juices from the kitchen counter and then wash your hands and dry them on that same towel. Or the towel falls on the floor after you wipe up the raw meat juices, and you forget which towel you had used and later pick it up to cover cooked food.

It may seem obvious that scenarios such as these have the potential for germs to contaminate other surfaces, and that people would avoid them, but they happen. Studies using hidden video cameras during food preparation—yes, such studies have been done—show people frequently making these sorts of mistakes. Another mistake is to touch your face as you cook; doing so transfers germs both from yourself to the food and from the food to you. As a parent, I know it is inevitable that you often have less time to prepare food than you would like, but try not to rush too much in the kitchen, because this is when people take shortcuts that increase the chances of food-borne illness.

Cooking Food

When it comes to microbes, well-cooked meat is safest. On the other hand, overcooked meat isn't ideal either, because overcooking can cause substances like heterocyclic amines to form, and these substances have the potential to be carcinogenic (cancer causing). Different types of meat, poultry, and fish have different pathogen risks. Many people prefer to eat beef or lamb that is rare or medium rare (red inside), but this is less safe from a microbial standpoint. *Never* serve ground meats that are not cooked through. Ground meat usually comes from several different parts of an animal (or several animals), and it passes through more stages of human handling, so it has a greater chance of being contaminated with germs. In barbecue season, there are always incidents of food-borne illness from undercooked hamburgers, so make sure yours are well done. Pork must also be well cooked so that the meat is white, not pink, because raw pork can transmit a parasite called *Trichinella* (more on this parasite in a moment). Raw poultry (chicken, turkey) often carries *Salmonella* and must be well cooked so that the juices are clear and not pink. Stuff a turkey just before you roast it, so that germs inside the bird do not have time to multiply before cooking.

Fish should be cooked right after you take it out of the refrigerator. Bacteria can grow in fish that warms to room temperature before cooking, and a toxin called histamine can also be produced. Histamine, which can cause scombroid fish poisoning, is not destroyed by cooking. Fish with the greatest risk for histamine production include tuna, mackerel, bonito, albacore, and mahimahi, but all fish carry the risk.

Mussels have to be cooked and eaten on the day they are bought, and they must be kept on ice all the way from the store until the time they are cooked. Anyone who loves to eat mussels knows that they have to open during cooking and that the unopened ones should not be eaten. Recent studies, however, have shown that mussels can open in boiling water in less than one minute, but it takes at least one minute and as long as six minutes for their internal temperature to get high enough to inactivate viruses like hepatitis A and noroviruses that may have contaminated the mussels. So I recommend that you let mussels boil for about six minutes after the shells open. People with liver disease or with a suppressed immune system should avoid consuming raw shellfish (mussels, oysters, clams), because they have a high risk of developing severe disease from germs in these foods. Young children also should avoid raw fish and shellfish.

The best way to ensure that meat and fish are adequately cooked is to use a meat thermometer. Insert the thermometer into the thickest part of the meat and be careful that it does not touch any bone, gristle, or fat. (Remember to wash the thermometer with soap and water before and after each use.) The U.S. Department of Agriculture (USDA) recommends that food be cooked until it reaches the following internal temperatures:

- Fish, steaks, and roasts (including beef and lamb): 145°F
- Ground beef and pork: 160°F (reheat ground beef leftovers to 165°F)
- Chicken and other poultry: 165°F

A few other foods require mention as well. As with poultry, raw eggs can be contaminated with *Salmonella*; the risk is small but real. Avoid offering raw or lightly cooked eggs (boiled less than ten minutes) to young children. The same goes for homemade mayonnaise, ice cream, and other foods that are prepared with raw eggs.

Unpasteurized dairy products, such as cheese and milk, carry a greater risk of being contaminated with pathogens, so children should not eat these products. Unpasteurized fruit juices can be a source of food-borne germs as well. Children should drink only pasteurized fruit juices, with one exception: freshly squeezed juices from well-washed fruits are appropriate (and are rich in vitamins), but the juice must be consumed right after squeezing.

Storing Food

In addition to proper preparation and cooking, food must be properly stored—both before it is prepared and after it is cooked—to keep the microbes at bay. Room temperature promotes the growth of many germs, even in cooked food, as well as the germination and growth of spores from some types of bacteria. Keep all meats, fish, eggs, and dairy products in a refrigerator, which should be set to maintain a temperature at or below 40°F, or in a freezer, which should be at or below 0°F. Many vegetables and some fruits will also last longer if they are refrigerated, although their vitamin content (vitamin C and several of the B complex vitamins) decreases the longer they stay in the refrigerator before consumption.

Store perishable items, including eggs, in the main part of the refrigerator, not in the door, because the temperature fluctuates more for items in the door as it is opened and closed. In the refrigerator, make sure that raw and cooked foods are in different areas and that juices from raw meat do not spill onto fruits and vegetables that are to be eaten uncooked.

Leftovers should go into the refrigerator immediately after eating. Do not leave freshly cooked food to cool outside the refrigerator; wait until it is no longer steaming and then refrigerate it. By refrigerating food not intended for immediate consumption, you decrease the risk of microbes beginning to grow. The USDA Food Safety and Inspection Service (www .fsis.usda.gov) has more information about safe storage for many different kinds of food.

Cleaning Up

Germs love moisture, and kitchens have all sorts of damp surfaces where they can multiply. Studies conducted in home kitchens have shown that the highest germ counts are in the sink and on sponges and dishrags used for cleaning. When you use the same sponge in the sink, on dishes, and on kitchen counters, you carry germs from the sink to the other surfaces. Studies have shown that 15 percent of sponges used in household sinks have *Salmonella* bacteria on them.

Keeping sponges and dishrags clean is actually quite easy. Keep several dishrags on hand so that you can rotate among them, and launder the used ones every two or three days. Several years ago, a study in the United States showed that putting sponges in the microwave for two minutes sterilizes them. (But do not microwave sponges with metallic parts: when the study's results were first announced, there were several instances of short circuits and fires caused by metallic cleaning items being heated in microwaves.) Wooden cutting boards (but not plastic ones) can also be disinfected safely in a household microwave. Plastic cutting boards are best cleaned in a dishwasher.

When washing up and cleaning the kitchen after food preparation, it is a good practice to dry washed items. This goes for kitchen counters as well as for dishes and silverware.

Grocery Shopping: Avoiding Germs at the Supermarket

If your children are like mine, they want to touch everything. This behavior is completely normal: children learn about and explore their environment and the wonders it contains using all their senses, touch included. Because children often bring their hands to their mouths, they can easily transmit germs from the surfaces they touch.

In food stores, raw meats are the most likely foods to be carrying germs. Studies of commercially available meats in the United States have shown that at least 20 percent, and perhaps as much as 70 percent, of poultry is contaminated with *Campylobacter,* and at least 20 percent of ground meat (chicken, turkey, pork, and beef) is contaminated with *Salmonella.* Therefore, you should be especially vigilant near the meat counter and not let your children touch meat or even the ice where meat is displayed. If your child is small enough to be in a stroller or store cart, then position her where she cannot reach any meat displays. If your child is older, take the time to explain that only you will handle the meat packages and that she can help you in other parts of the store. Also keep your eye on the supermarket or butcher shop employees; they should not touch meat with their bare hands. In fact, anyone in the store who handles unpackaged foods like bread, cookies, and other baked goods or who prepares sandwiches and deli items needs to wear gloves.

When buying any perishable item—and for that matter, nonperishable foods—check the expiration date or best-before date. If the date has passed, do not buy the product. Also avoid buying foods, such as milk, yogurt, and other dairy products, with broken, swollen, corroded, or otherwise altered packaging. These packages now have a pathway for germs to get into the food, where they can multiply.

The handles of food store carts are great places to find germs. Studies have shown that cart handles can have more germs than public toilets—incredible but true. Some food stores in the United States have started to offer sanitizing tissues to clean cart handles. Make use of these if they are available where you buy groceries, especially if you are placing a baby or toddler in the cart.

Packing the groceries into bags to carry home requires some thought as well. Food store employees should know that raw meat, fish, and poultry must be placed in a different bag from baked goods, fresh produce, chocolate, and any other foods that will be consumed without further cooking. When you get home, place the meat in the freezer or refrigerator right away.

Try to plan your shopping so that you buy your groceries last before returning home. Take them straight to your home and refrigerate them immediately. If it will take you longer than one hour to return home from the grocery store, use a cooler or insulated grocery bag for perishable items. And remember that reusable grocery bags can also be contaminated with bacteria, as a recent study showed. Always place raw foods in a separate bag and wash or bleach your reusable grocery bags regularly, particularly if they have been used to carry raw meats, fish, or poultry.

Eating Out: Think Before You Order

Eating out is fun and exciting for children, and you want it to stay that way rather than become associated with memories of food poisoning. The first rule to remember is the basic one that I will repeat several times throughout this book: before eating out, wash your own hands and have children wash their hands. When you are deciding where to eat, choose a reliable venue, particularly for children. Be especially wary when buying food from street vendors.

Avoid certain foods altogether, especially for children. Children should not eat raw shellfish or unpasteurized dairy products such as cheese—even if you personally know the cheese maker. Sprouts have been associated with many diarrheal outbreaks, so it is safest to avoid them on your children's sandwiches or salads. Ensure that foods like ground meat, poultry, and fish have been thoroughly cooked before your children begin eating. Cooked food should be eaten when it is still very warm; if it is served to you when it is still too hot to eat, you can assume that it is safe. And use your eyes and nose: if food has a suspicious color or smell, simply do not eat it.

In some places, especially many African, Asian, and South American countries, the water might not be clean, so use the general rule with food to "cook it, peel it, or forget it" in such settings. Therefore, you should avoid raw vegetables, salads, and fruit unless you have peeled them yourself (with clean hands). If water quality is not guaranteed, do not drink tap water; ask for drinks without ice added, because the ice will most likely have been made from the unclean tap water. In chapter 6, I give more details about food and drinks while traveling.

Exotic Cuisines

Many people, myself included, love eating the cuisine of other nations. But along with more opportunities to taste new flavors and exotic foods, there are more opportunities to ingest food-borne germs and sometimes to contract unusual diseases.

As an example, let's take sushi, one of the best-known exotic cuisines, which is now widely available in the United States. Sushi has spread beyond Japanese restaurants to many supermarkets and deli counters. My son was asking for it when he was only six! Sushi, which comes from Japan and Korea, is made from very fresh raw fish, rice, pickled and raw vegetables, and various condiments. Raw fish can transmit many germs, mainly bacteria and viruses that are in water. In addition, both freshwater and salt water fish may be colonized by parasites that can be transmitted to humans unless they are destroyed by freezing or thorough cooking. In the United States, the risk of a parasitic infection from raw or undercooked fish is relatively low, but it is still worth knowing the risks and how to minimize them.

A parasite called *Anisakis,* found in salmon, cod, sole, octopus, squid, herring, mackerel, flounder, and other kinds of fish, has the potential to cause serious disease. Symptoms start 1 to 24 hours after eating raw or undercooked fish and typically include sudden abdominal pain accompanied by vomiting and fever. Deep freezing (–31°F) raw fish for at least 48 hours before preparing sushi destroys the *Anisakis* parasite, but it does not destroy others.

Gnathostoma is not killed by freezing. This parasite, found in carp, ice fish, loach, and frog, can also cause intense gastrointestinal symptoms and sometimes chronic symptoms such as weight loss and abdominal pain. Illness from *Gnathostoma* has not been reported in North America, but cases have occurred in Japan, India, Latin America, and the Middle East.

Another fish parasite, *Diphyllobothrium latum,* can be found in salmon, perch, trout, and other freshwater fish, primarily in alpine lakes, in the Danube and other regions of Europe, but also in Asia and South and North America, including in Alaska salmon. Consumption of raw fish contaminated with *Diphyllobothrium* can cause anemia, gastrointestinal symptoms, and weight loss. You can prevent all parasite infections by thoroughly cooking fish to an internal temperature of 140°F, a temperature generally exceeded by normal cooking methods.

Sushi lovers know that a particular kind of fish, the puffer fish, is poisonous, and that its toxin can cause nausea; neurological symptoms such as numbness or tingling of the lips, tongue, hands, and feet; and ultimately paralysis of the respiratory muscles. Puffer fish are usually found in tropical seas, but they have made their way through the Suez Canal and have recently been found in the South Mediterranean.

More frequently than parasites, raw and undercooked fish can harbor some of the viruses and bacteria that I described earlier in this chapter, including the hepatitis A virus, noroviruses, and *Vibrio* bacteria. In many parts of the world, lemon juice is used in various foods, especially with fish and raw shellfish, to enhance the taste. This practice may well have spread for its antimicrobial value, because the acid in the lemon juice reduces the risk of bacterial food poisoning. It certainly may help, but it does not entirely eliminate the risk.

Young children (and the elderly) should not eat sushi or raw shellfish (mussels, oysters, clams). And older children and adults who want to satisfy their craving for sushi should consume it only from reliable venues. I give my son California rolls and other kinds of sushi that contain boiled shrimp or cooked salmon rather than raw fish. These alternatives are tasty and safe. Always carefully read the packaging to find out the contents of each kind of sushi.

Another raw seafood dish is a soup called ceviche, which originates from Mexico and is now on the menu in many restaurants that serve ethnic and fusion cuisine. Ceviche is a cold soup that contains raw seafood marinated in lemon or lime juice. The germ-related risks of raw seafood are true for this dish, too, so avoid giving it to your children and eat it yourself only at reliable restaurants.

One other raw seafood needs mention: raw oysters. People who eat raw oysters, particularly people with weakened immunity or with liver disease, are at risk of infection with *Vibrio* bacteria, a group of germs that can cause illnesses ranging from mild vomiting and diarrhea to a life-threatening bloodstream infection called septicemia. Cholera, which people tend to think of as a historical and exotic disease, is caused by one type of these bacteria, *Vibrio cholerae*. Other *Vibrio* bacteria are found in marine waters along the eastern North American and Gulf of Mexico coasts, primarily in the summer months. Lower concentrations exist along the west coast of North America.

Fish and other seafood are by no means the only sources of food-borne illness in exotic cuisines. Pork can transmit parasites, particularly *Taenia solium* and *Trichinella*, both of which can cause a generalized (whole-body) infection that includes the brain (seizures), muscles, and heart. *Trichinella* can also be transmitted from game, such as bear and wild hog meat, that has not been thoroughly cooked.

Beef is another source of parasites, especially *Toxoplasma* and *Taenia saginata* (the beef tapeworm). A common dish in French cuisine, steak tartare, is prepared with finely minced raw beef, egg, onion, capers, olive oil, and lemon juice. The French have a higher frequency of toxoplasmosis than people from other countries, in part from eating steak tartare. Toxoplasmosis is usually a mild disease, unless the immune system is not working properly, as is the case for people with AIDS or cancer, people who have had chemotherapy, and people who take steroids. In these cases, the disease can harm the brain, eyes, heart, and liver. Toxoplasmosis infection is also serious for a pregnant woman, with potentially devastating results for the developing baby. I discuss toxoplasmosis more in chapter 4, because cats are frequently carriers of the parasite. Infection with *Taenia saginata* often does not produce symptoms; if it does, they include abdominal pain, nausea, vomiting, weight loss, diarrhea, and passing worms in the stool.

In addition to parasites, raw beef may transmit several types of bacteria, including *Salmonella*, *Shigella*, *E. coli*, and others. As discussed earlier, these bacteria can cause serious complications, particularly in children, so the best way to avoid them is for children (but also adults) always to eat well-cooked meat, especially when the meat has been ground or minced.

In many countries, people eat more than just the muscle of animals. Offal—the internal organs of an animal—are considered delicacies in many cuisines. However, these parts can transmit diseases. In particular, beef and lamb offal, as well as wild hog, boar, and deer meat, can transmit the hepatitis E virus when not thoroughly cooked. Hepatitis E is particularly serious in pregnant women, causing gastrointestinal symptoms and severe hepatitis. Several years ago, the news was full of reports about bovine spongiform encephalopathy, or "mad cow" disease, which we now know can be avoided with appropriate farming practices. To reduce the risk of acquiring variant Creutzfeldt-Jakob disease (vCJD), the human equivalent of mad cow disease, the CDC recommends that concerned travelers to Europe and other parts of the world that had cases of mad cow disease avoid eating the brains of cattle or beef products such as burgers and sausages, or avoid beef altogether. However, the risk of contracting vCJD from eating beef is extremely low.

Cheeses made from unpasteurized milk are particularly popular in Europe as well as among cheese aficionados in North America. Many cheese producers believe that pasteurization affects the cheese's taste and aroma. Unfortunately, unpasteurized dairy products can be a source of many food-borne germs: *Salmonella, Campylobacter, Brucella, E. coli, Yersinia, Listeria,* and various mycobacteria (including the one that causes tuberculosis). Given the serious consequences of some of these bacteria, children and pregnant women must not eat unpasteurized dairy products.

Last, wild mushrooms, which are popular in many cuisines, are best left growing in the forest, unless you are knowledgeable about which ones are safe. There are many poisonous kinds—some of which mimic nonpoisonous varieties—that can cause severe disease or death.

Picnics and Barbecues

In summer months, many of us, especially children, enjoy going on picnics and having barbecues. Because of the outdoor element to picnics and barbecues, keep a few things in mind to ensure that food stays safe. Foods with high protein content (eggs, poultry, meat, fish, dairy products, custards, cream deserts, homemade potato and egg salads) are potentially dangerous. After preparation, these foods should be either kept cold (at or below 40°F) or kept hot (at or above 140°F). Temperatures in between this range are unsafe, because bacteria grow most rapidly from 40°F to 140°F.

Canned meat and poultry that will be opened at the picnic site and eaten right away are safe, as are fresh fruits and vegetables (washed well) and packaged cookies, bread, and crackers. Sandwiches should be wrapped tightly in a plastic film wrap and placed in an insulated cooler. All mayonnaise-based salads (potato salad, pasta salad) should be kept cool. Serve only the amount of salad that will be eaten within one hour and keep the rest in the cooler.

All meats, including hamburger patties, should be cooked thoroughly (see the temperatures recommended in "Cooking Food" above). Hot dogs should be cooked to an internal temperature of 165°F. When taking foods off the grill, do not put the cooked items back onto the same platter that was used for the raw meat. Similarly, do not use utensils that touched raw meat on cooked food. Raw meat should be packed separately from other foods in a cooler. Also, if you purchase take-out foods, such as fried chicken or barbecued beef, eat the food within two hours of picking it up.

Transport cold foods to the picnic in an insulated cold-storage container packed with ice or freezer packs to keep food cold. Do not overload a cooler, because this may make it more difficult for food to stay cool. If you are driving to the picnic on a hot day, carry the cooler inside an air-conditioned car rather than in the trunk. When you arrive, keep the cooler out of direct sun, and open it as few times as possible. Consider packing drinks in a different cooler so that the cooler with perishable foods does not get opened repeatedly.

Hot foods can be transported short distances right from the stove in insulated containers. A thoroughly cooked casserole will usually stay safe and warm if you insulate it well (use several layers of aluminum wrap, followed by a towel) and put it at the bottom of an insulated container or box. Serve hot food soon after you reach your destination. For longer trips, hot foods need to be refrigerated at or below 40°F and reheated just before eating.

If you were gone for no more than four to five hours and your perishable food items were kept on ice, except when cooked and served, you should be able to save the leftovers. Fruit that is cut (apples, watermelon, and so on) should also be treated as perishable and eaten within one to two hours of being at room temperature. If there is any doubt, discard food rather than risk becoming ill.

Feeding Baby: Keeping Your Infant Safe from Germs

Feeding your baby can be a wonderful, sometimes frustrating, and always messy affair. Today's parents have more options available than our own parents did when they had to prepare everything themselves. Many parents still prepare their baby's food at home, and in this case, it is important to follow the same basic rules of kitchen hygiene that I described earlier. Increasingly, parents are turning partly or completely to premade baby foods. The wide availability of foods from commercial companies has made feeding your baby easier, especially if you are busy or traveling.

Premade baby foods are safe for your baby, because baby food production must follow strict regulations. In addition, baby foods have been enriched with vitamins and trace elements, but you should always read the label to find out what the food contains to avoid unnecessary additives. This is not to say that it is impossible for baby foods to be contaminated during their preparation, but the strict regulations in the United States, Canada, and European countries offer a very high level of security. When you buy baby foods, always check the expiration date. Store the containers in a cool place where they will not be subjected to large fluctuations in temperature, and throw away any foods with suspicious or unusual color, odor, or appearance.

Some foods are not suitable for babies because they have a high risk of being contaminated by germs. Do not feed your baby honey or homemade canned foods before she reaches one year of age. These foods can contain spores of the bacterium *Clostridium botulinum,* which cause botulism, a serious illness that can result in muscle paralysis in babies.

Food that has been half-eaten by a baby or bottles of partially consumed milk should be discarded. Germs and enzymes from the baby's saliva can contaminate or alter the remaining food, so it is better not to keep them, even in the refrigerator. You should also avoid putting your baby's spoon, fork, or cup in your own mouth, because an adult's mouth has a lot of bacteria and viruses that could be transmitted to your vulnerable baby. Never place a pacifier in your mouth either. I have seen parents pick a baby's fallen pacifier off the floor, place it in their own mouth to "clean off" the germs, and give it back to their baby. In reality, these parents add to or replace the germs on the pacifier with their own mouth germs. Similarly, it is not a good idea for parents to premasticate (prechew) their baby's food in their own mouth before giving it to the baby.

Some of the germs that parents may pass from their mouth to their baby's mouth can cause long-term conditions. For example, *Helicobacter*

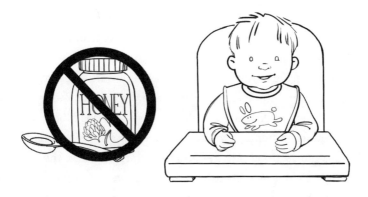

pylori is a bacterium that can lead to gastritis and stomach ulcers. Other examples are the hepatitis B virus, which can cause liver disease and cancer later in life, and the herpes virus, which can cause cold sores on the lips. Even HIV has been transmitted to babies from caregivers who were HIV infected and gave the baby premasticated food—the HIV was in blood present in the caregiver's saliva! Keep a second pacifier available to give your baby and rinse the pacifier that fell on the ground really well under running water. Periodically place the pacifier in boiling water for five minutes. (Be careful after boiling a pacifier that it is not hot when you give it back to your baby, and remember to empty any hot water from inside the nipple.)

The safest way to wash a baby's bottles to remove germs is to use a dishwasher with hot water and a warm-air drying cycle. If you wash baby bottles by hand, use warm water and soap and rinse them very well with water. Ideally, place hand-washed bottles in a moderate oven (about 250°F) for twenty minutes or in a microwave oven for four minutes to eliminate any germs that survived hand washing.

Children are more likely than adults to have symptoms from gastrointestinal infections, and symptoms are typically more severe. Children suffer more from loss of fluids and become dehydrated both more easily and more quickly. However, antiperistaltic drugs for diarrhea should be avoided in children younger than two years of age and in people of all ages who have fever and bloody diarrhea, because these drugs delay the body's responses to remove the germs and their products from the gastrointestinal tract. Gastrointestinal symptoms from food poisoning usually clear up if the child avoids eating for a few hours and, as soon as the vomiting stops, takes sips of liquid to replace lost fluids. Good sources of fluid replacement are Pedialyte, Ricelyte, and, for an older child, drinks such as Gatorade. If gastrointestinal symptoms are still present after three or four hours in an infant younger than one year old or after six to eight hours in an older child, or if the child appears ill or has bloody or unusually severe diarrhea, contact your pediatrician for further guidance.

Several organizations provide current information on their websites about food-borne diseases, including the CDC (www.cdc.gov/foodnet and www.cdc.gov/foodsafety) and the Partnership for Food Safety Education (www.fightbac.org).

───────────────────┤ MAIN POINTS ├───────────────────
Measures to Avoid Food Poisoning

- Wash your hands before preparing food, before eating food, and after using the toilet.
- Carefully clean food preparation surfaces.
- Wash fresh fruits and salad vegetables.
- Thoroughly cook meats, particularly all ground meats, pork, and chicken.
- Avoid giving raw fish and shellfish, raw eggs, and unpasteurized milk and dairy products to young children.
- Vaccinate your children against hepatitis A.

2

A, B, C and 1, 2, 3

COMMON GERMS AT DAY CARE AND SCHOOL

Many children spend substantial time at day care or at school. Often, both parents work outside the home, so more than two-thirds of children younger than six years attend a day care. Typically, a child today is exposed to other children in a group setting at a younger age than several decades ago, which has many positive aspects for a young child, such as learning social skills at a younger age. In many cases, children begin educational activities and group play at younger ages, too. However, close contact with many other young children also results in more intense exposure of infants and young children to germs. Infants and toddlers are at particular risk of contracting infectious diseases from other children because they frequently put their hands and toys in their mouth, and they share toys with each other.

In this chapter, I discuss the germs and infectious diseases that your children are most likely to encounter at day care and school, how they are transmitted, and the most effective prevention measures. I also briefly describe symptoms and when to keep a sick child at home. Last, I give some advice about selecting a day care with good hygienic practices.

Runny Noses and Upset Tummies: Typical Infections at Day Care and School

Nearly every kind of infection—respiratory, gastrointestinal (of the digestive system), skin, eye, and others—can be spread in a day care, school, or other group setting, such as an indoor play park. You cannot always prevent your children from becoming ill with some of these infections.

Children who attend day care are often sick with respiratory or gastrointestinal illnesses, particularly during their first year at day care. In subsequent years, however, these children seem to have fewer respiratory infections, as well as a lower frequency of asthma and other allergic conditions. For example, most children will have six to ten colds a year during their first year of attending day care. Having this many colds does not mean that your child's immune system is weak. It simply means that he has had limited exposure to germs and is susceptible to new ones that he has not encountered before.

The frequency of colds decreases with time and with exposure to other children. Children ages 3 to 4 generally have about five colds per year, children ages 5 to 9 have three or four, and older children and adults have two or three. Episodes of diarrhea average one or two per year for children who attend day care. So do not feel guilty if your children go to day care. Studies have shown that children who stay home until kindergarten are subject to more infections and school absences during the first few school years because they are finally exposed to all the germs they avoided earlier. Of course, at this point a child can handle germs better than as an infant.

It is nevertheless worth taking whatever precautions you can to avoid your children becoming ill unnecessarily. One crucial thing that you can do to protect your children from contracting ear infections or from having a serious case of the flu is to not smoke. Children should not be exposed to secondhand smoke or even thirdhand smoke (smoke residue that lingers in clothing, upholstery, carpets, and so on). Another easy but effective measure you can take is to get into the habit of washing your children's hands, and then your own, when you pick them up from day care or school at the end of the day. If soap and water are unavailable or impractical, keep sanitizing hand gel, foam, or tissues in your car or bag.

The risk of infections at day care and school is not limited to children. Day-care employees and parents of children at day care have a higher risk than other adults of contracting infections from children. Some infections, like influenza, parvovirus, and cytomegalovirus, all of which I discuss later in the chapter, have serious consequences for people with suppressed immune systems, such as people with HIV or undergoing chemotherapy, and for pregnant women. If you have a suppressed immune system or are pregnant, take extra precautions, especially around people who are sick with the flu. For example, avoid taking care of a sick child or adult, or if you must, wear a mask. Do not reuse the mask. Throw it out immediately after use and wash your hands after removing it.

Respiratory Infections

Respiratory infections, which affect the lungs and airways, are the most common infections children encounter in group settings, both at day care and at school. Children younger than two years have a higher risk of getting respiratory infections if they attend day care compared with children of the same age who are looked after at home. For example, a child at day care will have almost twice as many colds and ear infections and a nearly ten times greater chance of getting pneumonia (a lung infection). The risk is less at day-care facilities with fewer children and increases in proportion to the number of children who share the same room.

The germs responsible for respiratory infections in children are the same ones that circulate in the general community at any particular time. They include rhinoviruses, adenoviruses, respiratory syncytial virus (RSV), influenza viruses, parvovirus B19 (the virus of fifth disease), the bacterium *Pneumococcus*, and others. (These infections are discussed later in this chapter.) Many of the respiratory viruses contain hundreds of subcategories. For example, there are over one hundred species of rhinovirus, which cause the common cold. When a child comes down with a cold caused by one rhinovirus species, he builds immunity to that species but not to the remaining species. Because children (and adults) remain susceptible to all the virus species they have not had, they can contract more than one respiratory illness even in a single season.

Respiratory viruses are highly contagious. They are transmitted from person to person through droplets that contain the virus when someone coughs or sneezes. A cough or sneeze can propel droplets as far as three feet, where they land on desks, books, toys, hands, faces, and any other object. Many viruses can survive more than thirty minutes, and some, like influenza viruses, for several hours on doorknobs, taps, books, toys,

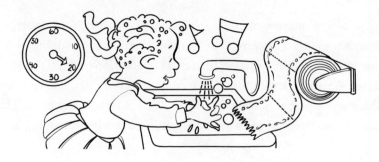

and other surfaces. It is not surprising, then, that when children return to group settings at the beginning of the school year or after winter break, they often get a cold within a few days. In fact, the well-known seasonality of respiratory infections may be more related to school schedules than to biological properties of microbes or outside temperature (although temperature and humidity do influence many viruses, such as influenza and RSV).

The spread of respiratory illnesses is difficult to contain among children, especially young children. However, it is never too early to start teaching children practices that limit the frequency of getting a respiratory virus. Frequent hand washing is essential, ideally with warm water and soap, although hand gels and foams containing alcohol work too. Everyone, children and adults alike, should wash their hands before and after they are in contact with a person with a respiratory illness, even a common cold. Children should begin learning how to properly wash their hands at about two years old. Proper hand washing means rubbing the palms, the backs of the hands, and all around the fingers with water and soap for about twenty seconds, or as long as it takes to sing the ABCs or "Twinkle, Twinkle, Little Star." After washing, hands should be dried well. I discuss hand washing and other hygiene procedures in chapter 13.

Another good practice is to cough or sneeze into your bent elbow rather than your hands, which then touch surfaces and leave the virus behind. Teach children to blow or wipe their nose with a paper tissue, immediately throw it into the trash, and then wash their hands. Adults who help to wipe a child's nose should do the same. It is also a good idea to avoid kissing children on the face when you or they are sick.

At least once every day, day-care employees should clean all surfaces, including toys, that children use. The cleaning procedure should include two steps:

1. Clean off visible dirt with water and detergent and rinse with water.
2. Sanitize with a household bleach solution from a spray bottle. Wet the entire surface until it glistens and leave the solution on the surface for at least two minutes before drying with a paper towel to give the bleach enough time to kill germs. Mix a fresh bleach solution every day with one tablespoon of bleach in one quart of cool water (or ¼ cup of bleach per gallon of water). Keep the spray bottle out of reach of children (even though household bleach at this strength should not be harmful for children if accidentally swallowed).

Any items that can be washed in a dishwasher or on the hot cycle of a washing machine do not have to be disinfected because these machines use sufficiently hot water for long enough to kill most germs.

Excluding or sending home a child with cold symptoms (cough, runny nose) does little to curb transmission of the virus to other children because a person is contagious with the virus for a few days before displaying symptoms. However, it is reasonable to exclude a child who has a fever or whose symptoms make him miserable enough to prevent participation in day-care or school activities. If possible, children with respiratory symptoms should be cared for in a separate day-care room; some larger centers have the capacity to do this. Day-care providers with respiratory symptoms should try to avoid taking care of children, especially young infants, and if they must work, they should wear a mask. In addition, infants younger than 3 months should not be in contact with either children or adults, at home or at day care, who have a respiratory infection.

Respiratory infections most often cause coughs, sore throats, and stuffy or runny noses. Typically, these symptoms are relatively mild and harmless, and they often resolve without treatment. Some parents may go straight for the medicine cabinet for antihistamines, decongestants, nasal sprays, and cough medicines to give to their children. However, these products are not effective at relieving the symptoms of a common cold in babies and young children, not even the products sold especially for children. In addition, they can have side effects such as drowsiness, irritability, and even breathing problems and seizures in young infants, so they simply should be avoided. The best treatment for a common upper respiratory infection in an otherwise healthy child is to let the virus run its course, which usually lasts for up to one to two weeks. Rest, liquids, and medicine to reduce fever, if necessary, are all a child needs.

Respiratory Syncytial Virus

RSV is very common in children and causes respiratory illness, including bronchiolitis (an inflammation of the small airways), and pneumonia, and may even lead to asthmatic episodes (wheezing). The illness sickens or kills many young children all over the world, and it is particularly serious in babies born prematurely. It also affects adults and can be serious in the immunocompromised and the elderly. The virus is spread through contact with secretions like droplets from coughs and sneezes, as well as from contaminated objects. RSV can persist on surfaces for many hours and for a half hour or more on hands. RSV occurs in annual epidemics during winter and spring, and it commonly spreads among household members and at day-care facilities, among both children and adults. Symptoms include those of an upper respiratory infection, with nasal congestion and cough, fever, lethargy, irritability, and poor feeding. Some patients with RSV infection experience wheezing and difficulty breathing or apnea (when breathing stops for a few seconds), particularly babies who were born prematurely, young infants, and people with heart disease or immunodeficiency.

The best way to prevent transmission of RSV is to administer a monoclonal antibody injection monthly during RSV season, beginning in early November, in selected high-risk infants and children (those with a history of premature birth, chronic lung disease, or congenital heart disease). If your child is in a high-risk group, your pediatrician will advise you about this injection. Where feasible, I recommend limiting exposure of high-risk children to contagious settings such as day-care centers. The risk of RSV transmission can be minimized with good hand hygiene. It is not necessary for a child sick with RSV to stay home from day care, unless he has a fever or requires more care than day-care providers can give.

Influenza

Influenza, commonly shortened to flu, is a respiratory illness that can be severe and often causes children to be absent from day care or school. It is frequently called seasonal flu because the virus strains typically circulate in communities between fall and early spring. Flu affects people of all ages, but children younger than two years and older adults are at higher risk of being severely ill with flu and are more likely to develop complications such as pneumonia; infection of the brain, heart, and muscles; and even death. As with other respiratory viruses, the flu virus passes from person to person through droplets or objects that have been contaminated with droplets. A child spreads the virus for at least a day before the onset of symptoms and for ten or more days after symptoms begin. The flu virus can survive for five minutes on hands, for eight to twelve hours on cloth or paper napkins, and for twenty-four to forty-eight hours on nonporous surfaces like tables, cups, and plastic or metal toys.

The best preventive measure against seasonal flu for children, day-care employees, parents of young infants, schoolteachers, and anyone for that matter, is to be vaccinated every fall. Annual vaccination is necessary because the flu virus mutates constantly, and every year the circulating strains are different from the previous year's. There are two kinds of flu vaccine: an intramuscular, inactivated vaccine for children 6 months of age and older and an intranasal, attenuated vaccine for children two years of age and older. Both vaccines are about 70 to 90 percent effective. In addition to preventing respiratory symptoms, the flu vaccine can decrease by as much as 40 percent the number of ear infections in people who receive it. When a child younger than nine years receives the flu vaccine for the first time, he should have it in two doses.

In addition to vaccination, the transmission of flu can be prevented with the same hygiene measures that apply for the common cold: frequently washing hands with water and soap or alcohol-based hand gels, and daily cleaning of surfaces and toys used by children. Dishes and silverware should be washed with warm water and detergent or in a dishwasher. In addition, towels should be changed frequently and washed in hot water in a washing machine; at day care and schools, it is preferable to use single-use paper napkins.

Crib or bed sheets and clothing, especially of a sick person, should be washed in the same way. When you do the laundry, avoid hugging the dirty items to your body as you carry them, and wash your hands after touching the dirty laundry. The influenza virus is destroyed at high temperatures (165°F to 210°F), and several chemicals, including bleach, hydrogen peroxide, detergents, iodine-containing antiseptics, and alcohol, are effective against the virus if they're applied at the right concentration for the right length of time.

Additional details about influenza prevention can be found on the CDC website (www.cdc.gov/flu). Boxes in this chapter describe pandemics in general and the H1N1 flu pandemic of 2009.

Fifth Disease

Fifth disease is a moderately contagious respiratory infection that often circulates in day-care centers and schools. It is caused by parvovirus B19 (which is different from the parvoviruses that affect animals, which you may hear your vet talking about) and is spread through coughs and sneezes as well as contact with saliva and the mouth. In a child, fifth disease usually begins with mild respiratory symptoms similar to a common cold; a few days later the child develops a faint, lace-like rash on the body and redness on the cheeks, commonly called "slapped cheeks." Once the rash has developed, the child is no longer contagious and can attend school or day care.

Infection in adults can cause joint pain, and in people with suppressed immune systems, the infection can cause severe anemia (a blood deficiency). Pregnant women who did not have fifth disease in childhood (and therefore did not develop immunity to the illness) are at particular risk because of problems for the fetus, which can include anemia, edema (general swelling), heart failure, and sometimes fetal death. Such serious problems in the fetus are rare, occurring in one of two hundred nonimmune pregnant women exposed in a day care and one in eighty nonimmune pregnant women exposed at home. Prevention is best accomplished through good hygiene and by teaching children not to share silverware and drink containers.

What Is a Pandemic?

The genetic code within flu viruses mutates constantly, so every year the main strains that circulate among human populations are different. The vaccines to prevent flu outbreaks must change too. Typically, genetic changes in the flu viruses are small from one year to the next (called genetic *drift*), which gives partial immunity to people who have been exposed to previous viruses or vaccines. Sometimes, however, a virus undergoes a large genetic change. In this case, the virus has changed significantly (called genetic *shift*), and people are now very susceptible to becoming ill from the new virus because nobody has protective antibodies against it. If the new virus has the capacity to spread easily from person to person, then conditions are ripe for a pandemic—a generalized, worldwide epidemic.

Pandemics of influenza have happened in intervals of ten to forty years (1889, 1918, 1957, 1968, and 2009). Every one of these pandemics developed suddenly, and each virus that caused them was radically different from previously circulating viruses. In several instances, these pandemics started in China, with the notable exception of the 2009 H1N1 flu pandemic (described in the next box).

Sometimes, a pandemic-causing virus originates from a mixture of human flu virus and flu virus from another species, like birds or pigs. For example, in the late 1990s, a bird flu virus mutated, and humans became susceptible to contracting it from infected birds. This virus was the H5N1 subtype, which caused panic but did not develop into a pandemic because human-to-human transfer is very difficult. However, scientists and physicians are carefully tracking this virus because of the concern that it will mutate again and cause a pandemic. I describe the H5N1 flu outbreak in greater detail in chapter 4.

Pertussis

Pertussis, or whooping cough, which is caused by the bacterium *Bordetella pertussis*, is on the rise in the United States, particularly in babies younger than 12 months who have not yet received all doses of the vaccine. Children who have not been immunized and adolescents and adults

The H1N1 Influenza Pandemic in 2009

In April 2009, international attention was drawn to Mexico, where a new strain of influenza virus had appeared, although there might have been earlier cases in the United States. It was an H1N1 type, which is a subtype of influenza A virus, and it contained parts from human, swine, and avian flu viruses. The new virus received several names: novel flu, new H1N1 flu, and new swine flu.

Being easily transmitted from human to human through droplets from coughing and sneezing, the virus spread quickly to the United States, Canada, Europe, Asia, and the rest of the world. It mainly affected younger individuals (5 to 24 years old), and unlike with seasonal flu, adults older than 64 years did not seem to be at higher risk of illness and complications. This unusual characteristic may be due to older people having partial immunity to the virus through exposure to previous viruses during their lives. Older adults are not necessarily immune, however, and they should still take precautions against getting infected.

The new H1N1 virus caused a high degree of anxiety internationally. The World Health Organization (WHO) declared a pandemic, and the virus's activity continued to be closely monitored. The CDC estimated that from April 2009 (when cases began to occur) to April 2010, between 43 and 88 million cases of new H1N1 flu occurred in the United States. The range is so large because people with milder illness tend not to seek medical help and therefore are not recorded.

who have not received a booster in many years are also vulnerable to pertussis. Infants may not have the typical whooping cough symptom of pertussis; rather, their symptoms may be a prolonged and persistent cough that can lead to gagging, vomiting, gasping, and even apnea (when the baby stops breathing for a few seconds). All children should be vaccinated, and all adolescents (and adults up to age 64 who are in contact with an infant or a patient with pertussis) should get one booster shot containing the acellular pertussis vaccine.

When an individual becomes sick with the new H1N1 flu, he can transmit the virus to others starting from a day before and up to five to seven days after symptoms begin—longer for children and patients with suppressed immune systems. As always, good personal hygiene habits are necessary to minimize the spread of the new H1N1 flu. During a pandemic, it's also wise to avoid crowded places and, as much as possible, avoid close contact between your children and other children.

There is a realistic risk that the virus could mutate into a more severe strain or into a strain resistant to antiviral drugs. The newer antiviral drugs against influenza (oseltamivir, zanamivir) have been effective against the new H1N1 virus, but they are most useful when given within the first two days after symptoms appear. Scientists worked feverishly to create a vaccine, which became available in October 2009. As with the seasonal flu vaccine, young children first receive the vaccine in two doses.

The symptoms of new H1N1 flu are like those of the previous seasonal flu: fever, cough, sore throat, nasal congestion, headache, muscle aches, chills, and a feeling of malaise or weakness. A substantial proportion of patients also develop vomiting and diarrhea. Serious illness and deaths have occurred, although the risk was not higher than the risk from seasonal flu. Almost 70 percent of patients who were hospitalized with the new H1N1 flu in 2009 and 2010 had a risk factor for severe illness, such as pregnancy, heart disease, asthma, diabetes, or kidney disease.

More information and ongoing updates about the current status of the new H1N1 flu can be found at www.cdc.gov/h1n1flu.

Tuberculosis

Tuberculosis (TB) is a serious infectious disease that most often affects the lungs. Although TB is rare in the United States, the number of cases has increased in recent years due to global travel; immigration from South American, Asian, and African countries where TB is more prevalent; and longer survival of patients with suppressed immune systems, who are particularly susceptible to TB. The mycobacteria that cause TB are transmitted through droplets when an infected person coughs or sneezes. Transmission happens from adult to child (or adult to adult) and not from child to child. Children can only rarely cough with enough force to expel the mycobacteria.

Day-care employees must be tested for TB before they start working with young children, particularly if they are in a higher-risk group. A few years ago, there was a TB outbreak at a U.S. day care, and nine children, all younger than seven years, were infected. The TB was transmitted by an adult employee who spread the infection to the children over a two-year period. Although the risk of acquiring TB at a day care is miniscule, the potential severity of the disease underscores the importance of every day-care center appropriately testing its employees to protect the health of the children.

Cytomegalovirus

Cytomegalovirus, or CMV, is one of the herpes viruses and is a common early childhood infection. It frequently infects children in day-care centers, where it is estimated that 10 to 70 percent of children younger than three years carry the virus at any particular time and secrete it in their urine or saliva without necessarily having symptoms. The virus can also be transferred to others from contaminated toys, surfaces like tables, and the hands of day-care employees. Basic hygiene practices are important, including washing hands, especially after changing a diaper, and cleaning toys and surfaces regularly.

Many children have few or no symptoms of CMV. Those who do may develop symptoms of a bad cold and fever for a few days or have swollen lymph glands in the neck area. In adults, pregnant women who are not immune from previous exposure to the virus are at greatest risk because the fetus may develop mental retardation, deafness, and vision problems. People who are immunosuppressed are also at greater risk from CMV.

Eye, Ear, and Mouth Infections

Conjunctivitis, or pink eye, is an infection of the outer surface of the eye and the inside of the eyelid. Viruses, bacteria, or allergies can cause it.

The viral and bacterial infections are easily spread from child to child, both in day care and in school, through person-to-person contact and from contaminated objects. Allergic conjunctivitis is not contagious. Transmission of a pink eye infection can be limited by practicing very good hygiene, including frequent hand washing and cleaning of toys, furniture, and other surfaces such as doorknobs and telephones. Also, children should not share towels. A child who has infectious pink eye with secretions should stay at home.

Ear infections can be caused by viruses or bacteria and occur most frequently in children younger than two years. Even though ear infections are not contagious themselves, they often follow an upper respiratory infection, and the bacteria and viruses that led to them can be contagious and are frequently found in children who attend day care. Therefore, good hygiene practices are necessary to minimize the chances of ear infections in young children. In addition, vaccination against *Pneumococcus*, a bacterium that frequently causes ear infections, has decreased dramatically the instances of ear infection and pneumonia in children. This vaccine is recommended for all children in the United States. The flu vaccine also reduces the risk of ear infections.

Ear infections cause pain and sometimes a fever, but the child need not stay home from day care unless he has a fever and bad respiratory symptoms or is very uncomfortable. Ear infections are often treated with antibiotics—in fact, ear infections are the main reason that small children receive antibiotics—but this treatment is not always appropriate. The inappropriate use of antibiotics, such as for viral infections, leads to antibiotic-resistant bacteria. I will discuss this issue in more detail in chapter 8.

Streptococcal pharyngitis and tonsillitis, commonly called strep throat, mainly affects school-aged children. It is caused by the bacterium *Streptococcus*, which can be transmitted from an infected child to other children or to adults through close physical contact or by sharing drink containers and silverware. Because the strep bacteria can remain alive on contaminated objects, you should change your child's toothbrush after his treatment for strep throat to avoid the chance of reinfection. In the rare case of a strep throat outbreak in a day care, all toys that children could have put in their mouths should be boiled or otherwise decontaminated.

A sore throat, fever, and headache are the main symptoms of strep throat, which is diagnosed by swabbing the throat and detecting or culturing the bacteria in a medical lab. A child with strep throat will be prescribed a course of antibiotic treatment and should stay home from school for twenty-four to forty-eight hours after starting the antibiotics.

Herpes infections of the mouth are caused by the herpes simplex virus. In children 1 to 4 years of age, who are usually infected with the virus for the first time, the virus can cause many painful blisters on the gums, a condition called *herpetic stomatitis*. Older children and adults tend to develop an ulcer, or open sore, on the lips (sometimes called a fever blister), particularly after a stressful situation.

The virus is very contagious and can spread easily from child to child or from adult to child through contact with the lesion or saliva—by a kiss, for example. The virus also spreads among athletes, particularly in sports like wrestling or rugby with physical contact between the players. To avoid transmission of the herpes virus, children should avoid close contact with someone who has a fever blister. Once a person has been infected with the virus, it remains in the body for life, so many people have the virus in their saliva even when they do not have a fever blister.

In most cases, a child with a fever blister can go to school or day care, provided that he avoids kissing and being in close contact with other children. However, when a young child gets a herpes mouth infection for the first time, called a *primary infection*, the symptoms are often severe (many sores in the mouth, drooling, and fever), so he should be kept home for a few days until the symptoms go away and he stops being contagious.

Hand-foot-and-mouth disease (HFMD), caused by an enterovirus, is another infection that can cause mouth blisters and sores, usually in young children. It is transmitted through contact with saliva and the mouth, including when children share silverware and drinking containers with each other. The best preventive measure is to teach children not to share these items. In a day care, employees should regularly wash toys that children put in their mouths. A child with HFMD should be kept out of day care, school, and swimming pools for the first few days of the illness.

Meningitis

Meningitis is a serious illness where the tissues covering the spinal cord and brain become infected. Meningitis can be caused by bacteria (such as *Meningococcus* and *Pneumococcus*) or viruses and is transmitted through droplets from coughs and sneezes or by close physical contact, including from unwashed hands or from sharing glasses or utensils. The risk of meningococcal meningitis is higher in crowded conditions, such as military camps and college dormitories, and may be slightly higher in day-care centers and schools. The risk of being exposed to viral meningitis, usually milder than bacterial meningitis, is highest in the summer.

If a child becomes ill with meningitis, the school or day care should be informed so that other parents are told. In some cases of bacterial meningitis, children who were exposed to the sick individual should take preventive antibiotics. The degree of risk depends on your child's association with the sick child, including how close their desks are. Your doctor can guide you appropriately if you are concerned that your child was exposed to *Meningococcus* or other causes of bacterial meningitis.

The symptoms of meningitis include headache, stiff neck, fever, vomiting, and heightened sensitivity to bright lights. Young children may appear to be particularly irritable and drowsy. If you suspect meningitis in your child, take him for medical attention immediately, because the repercussions of meningitis can be serious, sometimes with long-lasting effects.

A child with suspected meningitis is always given antibiotics until test results indicate the cause, because bacterial meningitis is serious and needs prompt antibiotic treatment.

Gastrointestinal Infections

Gastrointestinal infections, abbreviated to GI infections, involve the digestive system: the stomach and intestines. A GI infection is sometimes referred to as the "stomach flu," although the illness is not influenza. GI infections are caused by a wide range of germs, including viruses (for example, rotavirus, noroviruses, adenoviruses, and hepatitis A), bacteria (for example, *E. coli*, *Salmonella*, and *Shigella*), and parasites (for example, *Cryptosporidium* and *Giardia*).

GI infections typically occur because of food contamination and poor hygiene practices. These infections are more common in day care than in schools because children at day care are younger, many are not toilet trained, they frequently put their hands and toys in their mouths, and they share toys and other objects with each other. Acute infectious diarrhea is two to three times more frequent in children who attend day care compared with children of the same age who do not, and children are at highest risk of becoming ill during their first month at day care.

The chance of a child contracting a GI infection at day care depends on the number and ages of children at the facility, as well as the hygiene measures that are followed, in particular how frequently and how well the employees and the children wash their hands. Preventing the spread of GI viruses and bacteria requires careful hand washing and cleaning of potentially contaminated surfaces. Diapers and soiled clothes should be changed in spaces not accessible to other children, and these areas should have single-use paper covers or should be cleaned after each use. In addition, vaccines for rotavirus and hepatitis A virus are recommended for all children in the United States.

The main symptoms of GI infections are an upset stomach, vomiting, and diarrhea, and some people also have a fever. Children are at higher risk of dehydration, so a child with symptoms of a GI infection should be encouraged to drink fluids. A child with a GI infection will often pass it to other family members, depending on how strictly hygiene measures are followed at home. Of course, you should always follow good hygiene at home, not just when your child has a GI infection. With some infections, such as hepatitis A, children usually do not have symptoms, and the infection may not be discovered until a child transmits the illness to his parents. Adults can experience more severe symptoms from hepatitis A and may remain sick for weeks. Although hepatitis A was rare in preschool-aged children before the era of widespread day care, it has now become quite frequent among unvaccinated children.

Skin Infections

Staphylococcal skin infections, including boils, abscesses, cellulitis, and impetigo, are caused by the bacterium *Staphylococcus*. Staph skin infections were not commonly transmitted in day-care centers or schools until recently, when there has been a marked increase in these infections, which are frequently resistant to antibiotics (methicillin-resistant staph, or MRSA, infections). In the future, we may see even more of these resistant staph skin infections in day-care centers and schools because children share toys and other items, have close skin-to-skin contact, and are still learning about personal hygiene.

Impetigo, which can be caused by streptococcal as well as staphylococcal bacteria, appears as small red pimples with crusted yellow scabs, usually on the face. The infected area should be covered while the child attends day care or school; if it is impossible to cover the area, the child should stay at home until the infection has been treated.

Chickenpox is a very contagious infection caused by the varicella zoster virus. It can be transmitted through the air on dust particles and in tiny evaporated droplets, which can travel much farther than the usual three-foot span of a cough or sneeze droplet. Therefore, the virus can spread from room to room, floor to floor, and even building to building. Vaccination against chickenpox is the best prevention for this disease; the vaccine is 70 to 90 percent effective in preventing mild to moderate infection and more than 95 percent effective in preventing severe chickenpox. Children who receive the vaccine but still contract the illness are generally protected against severe chickenpox and its complications, so having your children immunized is worthwhile.

Chickenpox is recognizable by the itchy, blisterlike lesions that can occur anywhere on the body and head. The rash generally clears up on its own, but children with chickenpox should stay at home until all rash lesions have crusted over, which can take from a few days to two weeks. If a child has herpes zoster (shingles), he can go to school or day care if the rash can be covered well and the child does not open the bandage or touch the affected area. If these conditions cannot be assured, the child should stay at home until the rash heals.

Hair Infestations

Head lice are small insects that live on the hair, mostly in children ages 3 to 12 years. Although the lice themselves do not carry disease, they can be passed easily from child to child in day-care centers and schools. Despite what many people believe, having lice does not indicate poor hygiene, and getting lice does not depend on hair length or how frequently hair is washed or brushed.

Lice are transmitted through direct contact with lice-infested hair. They can also be transmitted on hairbrushes, combs, headbands, hats, and scarves, although these routes are less common, because lice that fall off hair are usually defective and cannot infect others. In general, children should avoid head-to-head contact with other children and should not share combs, brushes, hair accessories, or head coverings. Children with lice and anyone who has been exposed to them should receive appropriate treatment right away. Children can go to school as soon as they have received treatment. The school should also be notified so that other children can be checked for lice.

Blood-Borne Infections

The hepatitis B and C viruses and the human immunodeficiency virus (HIV) that can lead to acquired immune deficiency syndrome (AIDS) are all blood-borne germs. The risk of transmission of one of these viruses in a day care or school is extremely small.

Hepatitis B is a chronic disease that can cause liver cirrhosis and cancer in later life. A small number of hepatitis B cases are known to have occurred in day-care settings when an infected child bit another child or when blood or other secretions, such as saliva, of an infected child came into contact with the mucosal membranes (eyes, nose, mouth) of another child. Not many studies have examined this question, however, so the risk of a child contracting hepatitis B at day care is not known accurately. A vaccine against hepatitis B is available and is recommended for all children in the United States. If an unimmunized child is exposed to hepatitis B, he should immediately start the immunization series and should also receive an immunoglobulin specific for hepatitis B.

Hepatitis C infection also affects the liver and can have long-term consequences, including liver cirrhosis and cancer. The risk of transmission through a bite or exposure of the mucosal membranes is not known. In general, however, hepatitis C occurs very infrequently in children.

There are no known cases of HIV transmission at a day care, and the risk of transmission through a bite is small. In fact, because their immune systems may be compromised, children infected with HIV are more at risk from exposure to other children's germs than healthy children are to contracting HIV from an infected child.

All day-care centers and schools should follow standard precautions to remove blood and bloody secretions from the environment, regardless of whether an individual is known to be infected with hepatitis B or C or HIV. Bloody secretions should always be treated as if they were contaminated, which means they should be cleaned up while wearing gloves. I include detailed guidelines for cleaning up blood in chapter 3.

Day-care centers and schools cannot refuse admission to a child with hepatitis B or C or with HIV. The child's parents, together with his doctor, should decide if and which day care is appropriate and balance the risks and benefits of the decision.

Which Day Care or School Is the Right One for Your Child?

Selecting the right day care or school is extremely important to parents, because they want their child to spend his days in a caring, stimulating, safe, and, of course, healthy environment. You may have less choice when it comes to schools, but when selecting a day care, I recommend that you visit more than one facility. You should ask questions and observe their practices to be sure that the day care you select has the necessary licenses and follows appropriate hygiene and safety rules.

The American Academy of Pediatrics and the CDC have published guidelines that day-care facilities should follow. Individual states also have their own regulations about health and safety practices for day-care facilities. When you visit a day care, you should check several points related to hygiene and safety, including

- the experience and training of the childcare providers
- how many providers there are for the number of children who attend
- how often the staff wash their hands

- whether all infants sleep on their back
- whether parents are welcome to visit at any time of day and without warning

In addition, every day-care center and school should have written policies for

- handling particular illnesses in children and employees
- excluding (sending home) people who become ill during particular illness outbreaks
- required vaccinations before being allowed to attend
- personal hygiene measures for children and staff
- environmental sanitation practices
- hygienic preparation and presentation of food
- informing parents of children who might have been exposed to certain germs

Measures to Prevent Illness

One of the best things you can do to help keep your children healthy is to make sure they receive all the recommended vaccines before they start day care or school, as well as during their school years. Before the advent of vaccines, many infectious diseases were very common among children, but today they are largely—and for some diseases, entirely—preventable.

To decrease the risk of infections in day-care centers and schools, all children, childcare providers, and teachers should be vaccinated against measles, mumps, rubella, chickenpox, diphtheria, tetanus, pertussis (whooping cough), and polio. Children should also receive the vaccines against hepatitis A and B, *Pneumococcus*, *Meningococcus*, hemophilus influenzae, and influenza. All these vaccines are part of the recommended vaccination schedule, which I describe in more detail in chapter 9.

Even if your children have received all the recommended vaccines, several illnesses, as described earlier in this chapter, can still be acquired through contact with other children. Despite the seemingly high number of infections your children may be exposed to at day care and school, there are ways to decrease the spread of germs. Studies have shown that when improved hygiene measures were applied in day-care centers, the frequency of respiratory and gastrointestinal infections decreased. The use of antibiotics by children also decreased, and fewer children and parents were absent from school or work. The most effective way to promote hygienic practices is for teachers and day-care staff to be trained, preferably by medical personnel, about health issues and illness prevention.

Day-care centers and schools, especially schools that offer preschool and kindergarten classes, should take the following measures to prevent infections:

- Each room should have a sink, and there should be separate sinks for food preparation and for hand washing. Food should be prepared in an area away from toilets and diaper-changing areas.
- Toilets and sinks should be kept clean. Single-use paper towels should be provided to wipe hands after washing.
- Children and employees should wash their hands when they arrive, as well as after they use the toilet, change a diaper, help a child wipe his nose or mouth, take care of a skin scratch or injury, handle trash, or touch a pet. Hands should be washed with either water and soap or with gel or foam containing alcohol.
- Children should be taught to wash their hands after using the toilet and before and after eating.
- Children should not share cups, glasses, spoons, and forks with each other.
- All toys and surfaces that children use should be cleaned with a sanitizing solution every evening when children leave. In particular, all toys that infants and toddlers put in their mouths should be sanitized at least once daily. An effective sanitizing solution contains approximately one tablespoon of bleach in one quart of cool water, freshly made each day.
- Surfaces used for changing diapers should be sanitized (preferably with a bleach solution) after each use. Alternatively, they can be covered with a piece of paper that is changed after each use.
- All surfaces contaminated with blood should be cleaned immediately with a 10 percent solution of bleach (one part bleach to nine parts water).

- The facility should be ventilated with fresh outdoor air, and the temperature should be maintained between 65°F and 75°F during winter months and 68°F and 82°F during summer months. Relative humidity should be between 30 and 50 percent at all times.

Sending or Keeping Your Child Home

Sometimes it is obvious when a child should not be at day care or school, but the symptoms of some illnesses, especially mild respiratory illnesses, can be hard to judge at times. In some day-care centers, the employees call parents and ask them to take their child home in the case of cold symptoms or a fever. In others, they may keep sick children at the day care provided they do not have a fever. Some day-care centers have separate rooms and care providers for children with symptoms such as a cough, runny nose, or mild diarrhea, so that healthy children are protected from these illnesses.

As a parent, you should find out the specific policies at your child's day care or school. In general, however, you should keep your child at home if he has any of the following symptoms:

- Fever, lethargy (abnormal drowsiness), difficulty breathing
- Diarrhea
- Vomiting two or more times in the previous twenty-four hours, unless it is due to a known noncontagious condition
- Conjunctivitis (pink eye) with secretions
- Lice (unless appropriate therapy has been administered)
- Stomatitis (infection of the mouth) with many sores in the mouth and a fever
- Skin infections, until twenty-four hours have passed since starting appropriate therapy
- Strep throat, until at least twenty-four hours have passed since starting appropriate therapy

Measures to Avoid Infections at Day Care and School

- Wash your hands thoroughly and frequently. Avoid touching your eyes, nose, or mouth. Teach children to do the same.
- Cough and sneeze into a paper tissue or into your bent elbow. Put tissues into the trash immediately after use. Teach children to do the same.
- Do not let children share pacifiers, cups, glasses, spoons, forks, towels, or toothbrushes.
- Wash all surfaces that could have been contaminated, including toys, with warm water and soap or with a sanitizing solution.
- Do not smoke near children, and keep children and infants away from passive smoking.
- Wash your children's hands when you pick them up from day care at the end of the day, and then wash your own hands and turn the water off by handling the tap with a tissue. Alternatively, keep in your car or your purse sanitizing hand gel or tissues to wipe your children's hands when you pick them up.
- Know when to keep a sick child at home.
- Find out about a facility's hygiene policies and procedures before deciding which day care to place your children in.
- Be sure that your children receive all recommended vaccines and booster shots at the appropriate ages.

Swim, Ski, or Wrestle

GERMS ENCOUNTERED WHEN PLAYING SPORTS

A quote from the ancient Greeks and Romans nicely sums up sports: "A healthy mind in a healthy body." As parents, we all know how beneficial exercise and athletic activities are for the physical and mental health and development of our children. The benefits are diverse: socialization, healthy competition, development of physical abilities, avoidance of obesity, and simply good fun. However, there are also some hazards associated with sports activities, principally sports-related injuries but also the spread of germs and infectious diseases.

In this chapter, I describe the infections that children are most likely to be exposed to while they play sports. I also discuss two infections, HIV and hepatitis B, which cause a lot of parental anxiety, even though the actual risk of children contracting them through sports activities is very low. In no way am I trying to deter you from having your children participate in sports. Rather, I want you to be an informed parent, because knowledge about infectious diseases can minimize the risks and sometimes lead to outright prevention.

Common Infections That Parents Should Know About

In general, people who play sports, both children and adults, are healthy individuals with lower vulnerability to infections and a lower risk of serious complications from infections than other segments of the population. Many studies in adults have shown that regular exercise strengthens the body's immune defenses and decreases the frequency of upper respira-

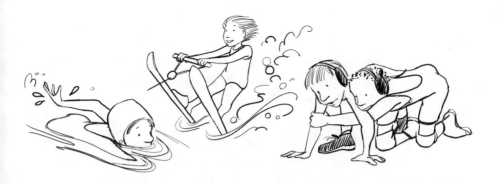

tory infections. Of course, moderation is the golden rule. Extreme stress, including extreme physical stress, makes the body more susceptible to infections. Indeed, many studies have reported that extreme exercise, such as training for a marathon, can lead to more frequent upper respiratory infections.

While participating in sports activities, people can spread germs in several ways. The main routes for germs to move from one person to another are through

- direct contact, meaning body-to-body touching
- indirect contact, meaning touching contaminated objects, towels, or clothes
- droplets from coughing, sneezing, or even talking
- sharing food or drinks
- the air

Infections can also spread among players or spectators at sporting events. For example, infections such as measles, chickenpox, and influenza can be contracted from airborne and droplet transmission of germs when playing or watching sports in closed stadiums with large crowds. The risk is lower when sports take place outdoors. The spread of these types of infections can be reduced if people get the appropriate vaccinations.

Skin Infections

Herpes infections, which are caused by herpes viruses, cause fever blisters on the lips (mainly herpes virus type 1) and genital infections (mainly herpes virus type 2). Herpes zoster, or shingles, is another skin infection that can occur in children (uncommonly) and adults (more commonly) and results from reactivation of the varicella (chickenpox) virus. These infections are transmitted directly through contact with infected skin and can also be transmitted indirectly through contaminated clothes or moist towels. Athletes who participate in sports with close contact have the highest risk of infection. The spread of herpes simplex infections has been documented repeatedly in high school and college students participating in contact sports like wrestling and rugby (the infections are sometimes called *herpes gladiatorum*). In addition, skin scratches and wounds may expose wrestlers to herpes viruses that may be present in their opponent's saliva or on the plastic mats on which matches are held.

To avoid spreading a herpes infection to others, athletes with symptoms of a herpes infection should avoid participating in their sport until the symptoms go away. Wearing clothes that cover the lesions might also decrease the risk of spread. Anyone playing a sport should take care to use only their own clothing, towels, and other personal items and not share them with other players.

Once a person has contracted a herpes virus, the body retains the virus for life, even though the person will not necessarily have symptoms. Herpes symptoms often flare up with any kind of stress, including injury, illness, psychological stress, menstrual period, or exposure to intense sunlight (ultraviolet, or UV, radiation). For example, alpine skiers are exposed frequently to a high dose of UV radiation because of the intense sunlight at high altitudes, and as a result they tend to develop fever blisters, especially during competitions when athletes are under stress. Preventive medications can be used to lower the chances of a herpes flare-up.

Warts on the skin are caused by human papilloma viruses (HPVs) and can be transmitted through repeated minor injury to wet or moist skin. For example, the soles of the feet are vulnerable to HPVs when walking on contaminated floors around swimming pools or showers, and the hands can come in contact with HPVs on contaminated gymnastics equipment or weights. The best preventive measures are to wear plastic sandals on swimming pool decks and in public showers and to use powder to keep hands and feet dry during gymnastics and weightlifting training and competitions. Warts can appear as rough, raised bumps on the

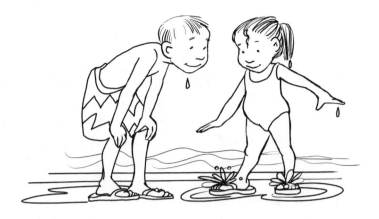

surface of the skin. Several products are available in pharmacies to treat warts, and family doctors have additional techniques they can use on stubborn warts.

Another skin infection that may be contracted from swimming in pools or possibly from sharing towels is *Molluscum contagiosum*, a common rash in childhood. The rash is caused by a virus and may persist for months. The lesions are pearly whitish and raised, often have a central pit, and can be anywhere on the body, but are usually on the face and hands. The lesions can be treated by removal, although usually this is not necessary because the rash will eventually go away by itself.

Bacterial infections of the skin, such as staphylococcal (staph) infections that cause boils, cellulitis, and other skin problems, are also spread through direct contact, particularly when there is a minor injury to the skin. Outbreaks of staph skin infections have been reported among schoolchildren who play football, rugby, wrestling, basketball, fencing, volleyball, and other team sports. To minimize the chances of being exposed to a staph infection, children should avoid sharing towels, ointments, creams, and lotions with other players. A child with a skin lesion should wear clothes that cover the lesion to avoid transmitting it to other people, or if it is difficult to keep the area covered, the child should not play sports with possible skin-to-skin contact until the symptoms of the infection have cleared up.

Symptoms of a staph skin infection vary and can include redness, swelling, pain, or warmth on the skin. These infections have become more difficult to treat, because staphylococcal bacteria have developed resistance to common antibiotics (methicillin-resistant *Staphylococcus aureus*, or MRSA). With antibiotic resistance, staph skin infections are a growing concern in schoolchildren and in sports teams in the United States, particularly because the infections take a long time to clear up and can sometimes be quite severe, spread to other parts of the body, and require hospitalization. Physical (skin-to-skin) contact, shared facilities and equipment, and hygienic practices of athletes all contribute to MRSA transmission among sports participants. Most reports of MRSA infections in athletes have been in football players, particularly in areas of injured skin (cuts, abrasions) and from artificial turf burns. In many cases, MRSA lesions are mistaken for insect or spider bites. To prevent MRSA transmission, teams should encourage better hygiene, including washing hands, using disposable towels, and sitting on a towel while on the bench; improve ventilation of showers and locker rooms; and clean facilities regularly. Teams should also routinely use sanitizers containing chlorhexidine or triclosan to sterilize wrestling mats and other shared equipment. Skin wounds should be covered during sports participation, and if the wound cannot be fully covered, infected players should abstain from competition until they have completed at least 72 hours of antibiotic therapy and remain free of moist or draining lesions. Coaches should also prevent athletes with open wounds from using whirlpools. I discuss antibiotic resistance in more detail in chapter 8.

A bacterial skin infection called *hot tub folliculitis* is caused by the *Pseudomonas* bacterium and infects hair follicles. The *Pseudomonas* bacteria are typically found in swimming pools, hot tubs, and spas, particularly when these facilities are used by many people and are not adequately cleaned. Outbreaks of hot tub folliculitis have also been reported from water slides, as well as in homes, related to bath toys and some synthetic sponges. Swimming pools and other aquatic facilities must be maintained appropriately, which includes monitoring water temperature, pH, and the concentration of chlorine and other sanitizing agents.

Hot tub folliculitis appears as a rash of red spots that may develop to look like pus-containing pimples. The rash may be worse in areas covered by a swimsuit, because these areas tend to stay wet with the contaminated water for a longer time. The rash usually goes away on its own, provided that it is not scratched, which can worsen and prolong it by allowing other skin germs to superinfect the area. (*Superinfection* occurs when a second infection, often caused by a different germ, develops in the same place as the first infection.)

Various species of fungus are also responsible for skin infections such as ringworm, jock itch, and athlete's foot. Fungal infections can also affect the fingernails and toenails. Fungi can spread from child to child through both direct and indirect contact in sports activities. Fungi prefer wet or moist places, such as sweaty skin, damp towels, showers, and closed sports shoes. To lower the risk of getting a fungal skin infection, children should avoid sharing towels and should use sandals to walk around swimming pools and gym showers. Pharmacies sell a range of over-the-counter creams and ointments that can be used to treat many fungal skin infections. Persistent infections of fingernails and toenails require a visit to a doctor.

Eye and Ear Infections

Conjunctivitis, or pink eye, is an infection of the outer surface of the eye and the inner surface of the eyelid that can be caused by viruses, bacteria, or allergies. Viral or bacterial conjunctivitis is very contagious and spreads easily by direct or indirect contact, as well as in swimming pools. To prevent its spread, a child with symptoms of pink eye (unless it is known to be from an allergy) should not play sports until the infection has cleared up. In particular, swimmers with viral or bacterial pink eye must not enter a swimming pool until the infection is gone. Typical symptoms of pink eye are pink or reddish eyes, itchiness, watering, and sometimes secretions that form crusts on the eyelids.

An outer ear infection called *otitis externa*, or swimmer's ear, is a common problem for swimmers, divers, and surfers. Swimmer's ear occurs when bacteria, typically *Pseudomonas*, infect the outer ear (the visible part of the ear and the ear canal). The outer ear becomes vulnerable to infection from extended exposure to water, which can irritate the skin in the canal and remove the ear wax. We have ear wax to keep debris and bacteria out of the ear canal, so without it, bacteria have easy access to infect the outer ear.

Children can minimize their chances of swimmer's ear by keeping their ears as dry as possible. When swimming or spending a lot of time in water, children can try commercially available earplugs to help keep their ears drier. Drying eardrops are available in pharmacies, but you can make your own by mixing together equal amounts of white vinegar and 70 percent rubbing alcohol. Put three to five drops of this solution into the ear canal after being in the water, but avoid using them if the ear canal is inflamed (it will sting). Symptoms of swimmer's ear include intense pain to the touch. Prescription eardrops may be necessary to treat the infection.

Gastrointestinal Infections

Infections of the gastrointestinal, or digestive, system such as gastroenteritis, salmonellosis, dysentery, and hepatitis have also been transmitted through swimming pool water. These illnesses are caused by various bacteria, viruses, and parasites, which I describe in greater detail in chapter 1. To prevent most infections from pools, swim only in pools that are well maintained with sanitizing chemicals and avoid swallowing pool water. In addition, young children with symptoms of a gastrointestinal infection, such as diarrhea, vomiting, or abdominal pain, should not be taken into a swimming pool.

Even if a swimming pool is adequately chlorinated, some germs, like *Cryptosporidium*, can survive and cause disease. Several *Cryptosporidium* outbreaks have occurred in the United States from contaminated swimming pools. This parasite can be removed from pool water with special filters, but not all pools have them. To prevent possible infection by germs in the pool water, children should avoid swallowing water when swimming in pools, keep their head out of the water as much as possible, particularly when the pool is full of people, and shower when they come out of the pool so that germs on their skin are mechanically removed by the water.

There have also been cases of gastrointestinal infections spreading among athletes from exposure to contaminated water, food, or drinks.

Respiratory Infections

Upper respiratory infections, such as the common cold, are caused mainly by a range of viruses. These infections are transmitted through droplets from coughs and sneezes, contact with the mucosal membranes (mouth, nose, eyes) of an infected person, and touching contaminated hands or athletic equipment. Children should be taught good personal hygiene and should avoid close contact with sick people to minimize their chance of contracting a respiratory infection. I discuss respiratory infections in detail in chapter 2.

Other Infections

Meningitis, an infection of the tissues covering the spinal cord and brain, is caused by bacteria or viruses that are spread by droplets or secretions from the nose or throat of an infected person. Typically, meningococcal meningitis, a bacterial form, is transmitted in places where many people live together, such as in college dormitories or military bases. There have been cases reported from crowding in dance clubs and bars, but not from crowds attending athletic events. Outbreaks of viral meningitis, which is usually less severe than the bacterial forms, have occurred in members of high school football teams.

Leptospirosis is a rare but potentially serious infection caused by the bacterium *Leptospira*. It can be contracted by swallowing water contaminated with the urine of infected animals (rodents or dogs). Most instances occur from swimming or doing water sports in rivers and lakes. For example, cases of leptospirosis have been reported in triathletes, who swim, bike, and run in the natural environment, and in kayakers, rafters, and swimmers. The symptoms of leptospirosis include fever with chills, headache, and a rash, and if it is not treated, the illness can progress to kidney and liver failure, or even death.

Infectious mononucleosis, often called mono, is a viral infection caused by one type of herpes virus. It is contracted from cough and sneeze droplets and from saliva (it is sometimes called the kissing disease). Mono does not usually spread among children in schools or on sports teams, but I mention it here because it tends to cause symptoms of fatigue, sore throat, headache, and muscle aches for prolonged periods. Therefore, athletes may not be able to perform well at their sport for up to three months after they have had a mono infection. In particular, it is important that intense sports and contact sports be avoided for at least one month after the illness starts, because of the risk of spleen rupture, even from a mild injury. Rupture of the spleen can cause a disastrous degree of blood loss.

Uncommon Infections That Parents Often Worry About

Although contracting a blood-borne disease while playing sports is extremely rare, many parents are concerned about the risks for their children. The human immunodeficiency virus (HIV), which causes AIDS, is frequently on parents' minds. HIV is transmitted from sexual contact and contaminated blood or needles, as well as from a mother to her baby during pregnancy, birth, or breastfeeding. To date, HIV has never been transmitted from one person to another through sweat, tears, urine, vomit, saliva, sputum, or respiratory droplets.

Because there is no vaccine or treatment to eradicate this virus, parents and students are often anxious about the possible spread of HIV while playing some sports, particularly sports like boxing or football, where the risk of getting an injury with bleeding is higher than in other sports. One study of American football examined the frequency of injuries that result in bleeding and the degree of contact between players and calculated the risk of HIV infection to be less than 1 in 85 million contacts during a game. In other words, a player is much more likely to become infected from having sex or using contaminated needles.

There is one case of a bodybuilder who was infected with HIV from intramuscular injections of anabolic substances that he performed with a needle previously used by an HIV-infected individual. A possible case of HIV transmission from sports contact occurred in an Italian soccer player who claimed he was infected after a bloody injury he sustained from a head-to-head collision with an HIV-infected player. However, his HIV infection was never proved to have been the result of this injury rather than other activities. Last, there are at least two reported cases of HIV transmission from fist fighting and resultant bloody injuries.

A second blood-borne disease that parents and players may be concerned about is hepatitis B, a chronic disease that can cause liver cirrhosis and cancer in later life. Hepatitis B is transmitted through the same routes as HIV (blood, sexual activity, and mother to baby). However, the hepatitis B virus is more easily transmitted than HIV. Transmission of hepatitis B has occurred among several members of a high school sumo wrestling team who sustained skin injuries during wrestling. In another case, five players on a football team contracted hepatitis B from injuries sustained during training. The best protection against hepatitis B is the vaccine, which is recommended for all children in the United States.

Despite the low risk of infection with HIV or hepatitis B while playing sports, athletes should take precautions when there is the potential of being exposed to blood. The American College of Sports Medicine, the American Academy of Pediatrics, the World Health Organization, and other associations have issued the following guidance for preventing infections that are spread through blood during athletic activities:

- An injury with skin penetration should be cleaned immediately with an appropriate antiseptic and covered for the duration of the match.
- An athlete with a bloody injury should stop participating until the wound has been cleaned and adequately covered. Blood-soiled clothes should be changed before the athlete returns to the match.
- Coaches should have first aid training and the necessary equipment to care for injuries. Equipment should include gloves, antiseptics, sanitizing solutions, gauze, and bandages, as well as the appropriate containers to dispose of contaminated objects, needles, or syringes.
- Athletic equipment and objects that are obviously soiled with blood should be cleaned and sanitized with a bleach solution before reusing.
- Individuals who take care of wounds should wear gloves if there is any possibility of contact with blood. Gloves should be changed after taking care of each athlete. Hands should be washed after gloves are taken off.
- Athletes who are infected with HIV should not be excluded from participating in sports unless other people are at substantial risk of exposure to their blood. Testing for HIV before sports participation should be strictly voluntary.

Measures to Avoid Infections while Playing Sports

- Don't allow children to participate in sports with close body contact (such as wrestling) or to swim when they have a contagious rash (such as fever blisters, chickenpox, shingles, or staph skin infections) or infectious pink eye. Young children with diarrhea should not swim either.
- Explain to children that they should avoid swallowing water in a swimming pool. Have children rinse themselves with fresh water when they get out of the pool.
- Have children wear plastic sandals or flip-flops when they walk around the swimming pool deck and in gym showers.
- Encourage children to avoid sharing cups, glasses, water bottles, bars of soap, creams, lotions, or towels with each other.
- Teach children to avoid contact with other people's blood.

4

Fur, Feathers, and Fangs

GERMS FROM PETS AND OTHER ANIMALS

People domesticated animals as pets and to help with farming and other work thousands of years ago, and we continue to have close ties to animals. Many people work directly with animals on farms, in zoos, at animal recovery centers, at animal training facilities, and so on. Living with animals is also common throughout the world. In the United States, nearly two-thirds of households have at least one pet, and many people share their homes with several animals. Typical pets in the United States are dogs and cats, and some people also keep fish, birds, rabbits, reptiles, and other creatures in their homes.

People may gain several health benefits, such as lower blood pressure and lower levels of stress, from caring for and exercising their pets. Pets can also provide companionship, not to mention the independence that many people are able to enjoy from having a trained guide dog. Naturally, there are some health risks too, which I discuss in this chapter. Children are often at greater risk than adults of contracting an infection from a pet because of the way children behave, both when interacting with an animal and when practicing (or not) good hygiene. As well as describing the possible infections that people can contract from living or working closely with animals, I mention a few areas of concern when people interact with untraditional pets or wild animals. In particular, I discuss rabies and avian flu.

Man's Best Friend: Pet Dogs

Considering the large number of households with pet dogs, the chances of dogs spreading diseases to humans are small. For a young child, the greatest risk from a dog is being bitten. Young children often play roughly and do not yet understand the necessity of being gentle around animals. For example, a child may simply want to hug a dog but actually annoys or startles it as it eats or sleeps. A new baby in a family can also become a dog's target, because the dog is unfamiliar with this new person and may feel threatened. The result of a family's dog attacking a child, whether a very young baby or an older child, can be frightening and devastating. In my pediatric career, I have seen several young victims of dog bites. Some bites have even caused skull fractures. A baby must never be left alone with a dog, and nor should young children be alone with a dog until the dog understands them and they understand how to interact appropriately with the animal.

Dogs (and cats, other animals, and even humans) have many different microbes in their mouths. Scientists would say that the microbial flora of the mouth is rich and diverse. Fortunately, many of these microbes do no harm to either a dog or a person who is bitten by a dog. The risk of infection after a dog bite is about 10 percent. (The risk is much greater from cat bites, which I describe in a moment.)

Immediately after a dog bite, the wounds should be rinsed well with clean water. A child who has been bitten should see the family doctor or a pediatrician the same day to have the wound cleansed properly and to find out whether he will need to take antibiotics. There are two schools of thought on whether to give a child antibiotics after a dog bite. Most doctors, myself included, recommend giving a child antibiotics as a precaution, particularly for wounds on the face or hands and for deep puncture wounds.

Sometimes a dog bite wound seems minor, and you may decide not to visit a doctor; in this case, keep an eye on the area over the course of the day. If, within hours of a dog bite, the area around the wound becomes red or swollen or shows any pus secretions, take the child to the doctor immediately to start antibiotics. This rapidly developing infection is usually the result of the bacterium *Pasteurella*. Infection with *Pasteurella* is much more likely after a cat bite, but it can also happen after a dog bite.

People who have a weakened immune system (from, for example, treatment with steroids, a blood cancer, an autoimmune disease, or other conditions) and those who have had their spleen removed should always be prescribed preventive antibiotics after a dog bite or even if they have an open wound that comes in contact with dog saliva. These individuals are at risk of a rare but very serious infection caused by *Capnocytophaga canimorsus*, a bacterium found in the saliva of dogs.

Tetanus and rabies can also be contracted from a dog bite wound; however, all children should have been immunized against tetanus, and the dog should have been immunized against rabies. Rabies in dogs is extremely unusual in the United States. Nevertheless, if there is any doubt about a child's tetanus or a dog's rabies vaccination, go immediately to a doctor for appropriate treatment.

Dogs may have parasites and other germs in their feces. For example, the bacteria *Salmonella*, *Campylobacter*, *Brucella*, and *Leptospira* and the parasites *Cryptosporidium*, *Giardia*, *Toxocara*, and *Echinococcus* can all infect dogs. Although uncommon, these germs can be transmitted to humans through the fecal-oral route (from the dog's feces to the person's mouth). Clearly, young children are at greatest risk because they frequently put their hands in their mouths and are still learning to follow hygienic practices. Puppies, particularly those younger than 6 months, dogs living in kennels or pet shops, and stray dogs have the highest chance of being infected with a germ that can contaminate their feces. For example, two intestinal germs, *Salmonella* and *Campylobacter*, have been found in over 30 percent of feces from young dogs.

Puppies with diarrhea and stray dogs should be kept away from young children and should also be avoided by adults who have a suppressed immune system. If you buy a puppy from a pet shop or adopt a dog from a kennel or shelter, take the dog to a vet for deworming. Someone with a weakened immune system who wants a puppy younger than 6 months should have the puppy's stool examined for the parasite *Cryptosporidium* before taking the puppy home. In addition, dogs should not be allowed to defecate at playgrounds, beaches, or areas of parks where children play.

If your dog does defecate in your yard, the feces should be removed at least once or twice a week. Dog feces (and cat feces) must never be used as compost.

Raw food diets for dogs (and other pets) seem to be the fashion these days. There are even commercially available frozen and freeze-dried raw food patties for pets. Proponents of raw food diets claim that eating raw meat and poultry is essential for the health of domestic dogs and cats and that it is microbially safe. Several research studies, however, have found *Salmonella* is common in the feces of dogs that routinely eat raw meat. Both dogs and cats can become ill after eating a *Salmonella*-contaminated diet, and even if they do not develop symptoms, they can transmit the bacteria to their owners.

The commercially available raw pet food products do not undergo safety regulations and often carry *E. coli*, *Salmonella*, and other bacteria. For example, a study found *Salmonella* in 7 percent of raw food samples available in the U.S. retail market and in up to 20 percent of Canadian samples. In addition, dogs should not be fed raw offal, because they can acquire the parasite *Echinococcus*, which contaminates the dog's feces and can infect herbivores and humans. The resulting disease, echinococcosis, is serious for humans.

Dogs (and other pets) are susceptible to having fleas or ticks in their fur. Fleabites are usually inconsequential for humans; sometimes they can cause a skin reaction with localized itching or a rash, both of which can be treated easily with antihistamines or anti-inflammatory drugs. Occasionally, fleas (or lice) on pets carry the eggs of tapeworms like *Dipylidium caninum*, the most common tapeworm of dogs, which can be transmitted to a child who swallows a flea by putting his hands in his mouth when playing with a dog. Most *Dipylidium* infections occur in children younger than 8 years, with one-third occurring in infants younger than 6 months. Rarely, dog fleas can spread diseases, such as typhus and other fevers, caused by *Rickettsia* bacteria, or even bubonic plague, caused by *Yersinia* bacteria. Dog fleas can be prevented and treated by spraying the areas where a dog sleeps or by applying special antiflea formulations on a dog's fur.

Dogs and other animals frequently have fungal infections like ringworm on their skin. Typically, ringworm infections cause a small bald patch on animals. People can also become infected with ringworm, with about 10 to 30 percent of these common rashes in humans probably coming from contact with animals. Children who pick up a ringworm infection may lose their scalp hair in one or more places or develop a round red rash on the skin. The fungal infection can be treated with a medicated ointment applied directly on the affected skin or with an anti-fungal medication given by mouth.

When a child has a ringworm infection, the home and other places that might have contaminated animal hair need to be cleaned carefully. A child with ringworm should not share hand towels and other such items with family members to avoid transmitting the infection. In addition, the family pet should be treated with an antifungal medication to get rid of the source of infection.

To be safe, teach children how to interact appropriately with dogs—with any pet for that matter. Children should learn to play gently with pets and not startle or aggravate them. They should avoid kissing an animal or getting their face too close to an animal's face. And when they have finished touching or playing with the pet, they should wash their hands well (preferably not in the kitchen sink, where subsequent contamination of food is more likely). Also, if an unfamiliar dog approaches, teach your child not to run away or act aggressively but to let the dog smell him and then slowly walk back while facing the dog.

Kitty or Tiger: Pet Cats

Cat bites cause infections more frequently than dog bites do. In fact, about 50 percent of all cat bite wounds become infected. Cats have smaller but sharper teeth than dogs, so a cat bite can penetrate the deeper tissues, such as tendons, bones, and joints. Preventive antibiotics should always be given after a cat bite that has penetrated the skin, and particularly for bites near joints on the hands, because infections near joints can become serious.

People can develop infections following cat scratches as well, because when cats lick themselves, they contaminate their claws with mouth germs like *Pasteurella. Pasteurella* can cause a serious infection, which develops within twenty-four hours of a bite or scratch and causes redness, swelling, and pain in the affected area.

Bites, scratches, or even just a lick from a cat can cause another infection in people, appropriately named cat scratch disease. This worldwide infection occurs mostly during fall and winter months and is caused by the bacterium *Bartonella henselae*, which occurs most frequently in kittens, stray cats, and cats with fleas (fleas can spread the bacterium from cat to cat). Children younger than 10 years old are the most likely to get cat scratch disease, and the risk decreases with increasing age. People with weakened immunity are particularly susceptible and can develop serious illness with cat scratch disease. Prevention includes treating your kitten or cat with sprays or other methods to prevent or get rid of fleas. If you have an immune-suppressed person in your family, discuss with a vet the possibility of culturing your cat's blood to find out if it has *Bartonella*. If it does, the cat can be treated with antibiotics.

Cat scratch disease typically causes a small lesion within one week of a bite, scratch, or lick. A child may not even remember having been scratched or licked. The lesion itself may also be so mild that it passes unnoticed. Weeks or months later, the child may develop swelling of the lymph nodes near the affected area, usually along with a fever. Rarely, the child can develop lethargy and seizures, enlargement of the liver and spleen, rashes, and bone infection. Although these symptoms sound serious, treatment is usually not necessary, because the symptoms go away by themselves, typically without long-term repercussions for the child. Some antibiotics may speed up recovery, which can take several weeks without treatment.

As with dogs, several germs, including bacteria (*Campylobacter, Salmonella*) and parasites (*Cryptosporidium, Toxocara*), can be present in cat feces and can be transmitted to people through the fecal-oral route. One additional parasite, *Toxoplasma*, is mainly transmitted through cats and can cause severe problems, especially for people with a weak immune system and for a pregnant woman's unborn baby. In any one hundred cats, only one will be infected with *Toxoplasma*, but this one infected cat will excrete millions of *Toxoplasma* eggs (called *oocysts*) in its feces for one to three weeks. The eggs can be transmitted to a person who cleans the cat's litter box or gardens in a contaminated area. People can also be infected in the same way that cats become infected: from eating contaminated meat, particularly pork or lamb but also beef that has not been well cooked.

People infected by *Toxoplasma* develop toxoplasmosis, a disease that usually causes few or no symptoms in a healthy individual. If a healthy person does develop symptoms, they may include fever, swollen lymph glands in the neck, fatigue, sore throat, and muscle aches, and they typically go away after a few days without treatment. Rarely, symptoms continue for a longer period. Also rarely, the retina at the back of the eye can be damaged, resulting in possible vision problems. People with weakened immune systems, particularly people on chemotherapy, can develop severe disease with damage to the brain, retina, heart, and liver. They generally need prolonged treatment.

When a pregnant woman contracts toxoplasmosis, even if she does not develop symptoms herself, the parasite can pass to the fetus through the placenta. The consequences for the fetus depend on the stage of pregnancy. Infection of the fetus during the first trimester is less frequent but can cause severe damage, including mental retardation, vision loss, jaundice (yellow color), and enlargement of the liver and spleen. As the pregnancy progresses, infection of the fetus becomes more likely but less severe. Infection near the end of pregnancy usually has no consequences for the fetus. Rarely, the child may develop vision problems many years later.

Because of the potentially serious consequences, pregnant women should avoid cleaning cats' litter boxes. If nobody else at home can take on this duty, the pregnant woman should wear disposable gloves and clean the litter box every day, because the oocysts are not infective during the first one to two days after they are passed by the cat. Also, pregnant women should not garden in areas where cats may have defecated and should avoid aerating rugs that may have been contaminated with cat feces. Last but not least, pregnant women should always wash their hands after petting a cat. (Unrelated to pets, but equally important, pregnant women who eat meat should ensure that the meat, particularly pork, lamb, and venison, has been well-cooked to an internal temperature of 150°F to 170°F and is no longer pink inside.)

Feathered Friends: Pet Birds

Birds do not spread many diseases to people. The most common disease that birds can transmit to humans is psittacosis, a form of pneumonia with a fever and a cough, caused by the bacterium *Chlamydophila psittaci*, which can contaminate a bird's feces. This illness is mainly a problem for people who spend many hours working with birds, such as on farms with turkeys, ducks, and geese. It occurs infrequently in owners of pet birds.

Bird feces may also contain some fungi, such as *Histoplasma* and *Cryptococcus*, which do not make birds sick but which can contaminate soil. If soil contaminated with one of these fungi is disturbed—for example, during building demolition—the spores of the fungi may become airborne and can be inhaled by people. Bats can also carry these fungi in their feces, so human exposure may occur in tunnels, caves, and mines where the soil is disturbed by human activity.

Usually people who inhale these fungi develop only mild flulike symptoms, but in people with weakened immunity, infection can be very dangerous, causing some forms of pneumonia or generalized disease (involving many organ systems).

Fins and Scales: Aquarium Fish

Disease transmission from goldfish and other ornamental fish species kept in an aquarium occurs only rarely. The main germs that aquarium fish owners may be exposed to are mycobacteria. Typically, mycobacteria enter a person through a skin injury when an aquarium is being cleaned. A mycobacterium infection can cause an ulcer (open skin sore) or other skin lesions, which may extend to deeper tissues. Someone diagnosed with this type of skin infection should destroy the infected fish and decontaminate the aquarium with a bleach solution before adding new fish.

Ideally, you should always wear long rubber gloves to clean a fish tank, and do not let children do the cleaning. Also, do not put the aquarium water in your bathtub; there was a case of a young girl who acquired a mycobacterium skin infection after taking a bath in a tub where the fish bowl water had been thrown out.

Other germs are rarely spread from fish to humans: divers and people who work with fish may get an infection after a skin injury from a fish.

Nibblers: Pet Rabbits and Other Rodents

Rabbits are some of the safest pets from the perspective of infections. They do not commonly bite, although they can scratch. It is possible, though rare, to contract the diseases mentioned for cats and dogs (for example, *Pasteurella*, *Salmonella*, and others) from a pet rabbit.

Other rodents, especially various kinds of mice and rats, are more likely to carry germs that can make people ill. Rat bite fever, a bacterial infection that causes fever, rash, headache, nausea, and joint pain, can result from a rodent's bite or scratch, mostly from rats, mice, and hamsters. Other illnesses that rats and mice can transmit are salmonellosis, *Pasteurella* infection (after a bite), leptospirosis, and tularemia, the last two being serious but, fortunately, rare. Mice and hamsters can also excrete the lymphocytic choriomeningitis virus in their urine and feces, and, rarely, this virus can infect humans. Infection by this virus is a risk mainly for pregnant women, because of possible miscarriage or problems in the fetus, similar to the effects of toxoplasmosis.

Sun Seekers: Pet Snakes and Other Reptiles

Turtles, lizards, iguanas, and snakes are all possible carriers of *Salmonella* bacteria, making salmonellosis the greatest risk from pet reptiles. As a pediatrician, I have seen enough cases of *Salmonella* infection in children to be convinced that reptiles are not suitable pets in homes with children younger than 5 years old. Toddlers do not follow hygiene rules to the letter, and as a result, they are not yet ready to take the necessary precautions to stay safe around reptiles.

Many outbreaks of salmonellosis have been caused by pet turtles. Turtles usually acquire the *Salmonella* bacteria from water ponds where they are bred, and they then become carriers and excrete the bacteria over many months. Turtle breeders used antibiotics in an effort to eradicate *Salmonella* in turtles but unfortunately caused an even worse problem: *Salmonella* that is resistant to antibiotics. The risk of *Salmonella* infection extends to other reptiles as well (and to other animals, including porcupines, amphibians [frogs, salamanders], rodents, and poultry).

Salmonellosis manifests with diarrhea, fever, vomiting, and abdominal pain, and it can cause severe illness in people with weakened immunity, babies, and older individuals. Because of the *Salmonella* risk, the Centers for Disease Control and Prevention (CDC) recommends that reptiles, amphibians, rodents, and baby poultry not be kept in households with children younger than 5 years, people with a compromised immune system, or people with sickle cell disease (a blood disorder). Because turtles are a major source of human *Salmonella* infections, regulations in the United States prohibit the sale of small turtles (shell length less than four inches), which children in particular may handle inappropriately and may even place in their mouth. This prohibition is not always enforced, however.

Less Common Pets: Monkeys and Other Animals

In the United States, laws restrict the importation of monkeys for the pet trade. These laws are medically justified. There are many reasons monkeys, and primates in general, should not be human pets. Evolutionarily, monkeys are close to humans, so many monkey diseases can spread to humans (see the examples in the box), and monkeys are also susceptible to human diseases.

Monkeys are frequently ill with the intestinal germs *Salmonella* and

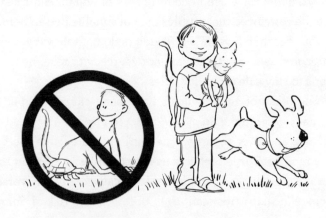

Wild Animal Diseases that Have Become Human Infections

All animals were wild at one time, and although some have been domesticated, principally dogs and cats, many other animals that people attempt
to keep as pets are simply not safe. In addition to the unpredictable nature
of many wild animals is the risk of new germs being introduced into the
human population, germs to which the human immune system is completely naïve. There are several recent examples of illnesses transmitted
from wild animals to humans.

First, the human immunodeficiency virus, or HIV, which causes AIDS,
was most likely introduced to humans via monkey hunters. A monkey retro-
virus that doesn't make monkeys sick adapted genetically and now infects
humans. The latest statistics from UNAIDS estimate that at the end of
2008, about 33 million people were living with HIV/AIDS worldwide.

Second, in 2003 in the United States, there was an outbreak of monkeypox, which causes a rash similar to smallpox, and ninety-three people became
ill. This outbreak was the first occurrence of monkeypox in the Western
Hemisphere. Despite its name, the illness was caused by pet prairie dogs
(which are rodents) that had been infected by African giant rats imported
to the United States to be sold as pets.

Third, also in 2003, there was an outbreak of a new disease, severe acute
respiratory syndrome (SARS), which spread from China to Canada and
many other countries. In less than a year, SARS had made more than eight
thousand people ill and caused over seven hundred deaths. It also resulted
in a lot of anxiety and disruption in air travel, tourism, and commerce. The
cause of SARS was a new coronavirus, which was introduced to humans
from an exotic cat species, the palm civet of the Himalayas, as well as from
certain kinds of raccoon in China. These animals had been sold as pets.

Two other infections—rabies and avian influenza—that humans can
acquire from animals are discussed elsewhere in this chapter.

Shigella, both of which they can transmit to humans. Monkeys are also
very vulnerable to respiratory infections, including tuberculosis, which
they can give to or acquire from their owners. They are very susceptible
to measles, too, which they can easily acquire from sick children. Some

monkey viruses are lethal for humans. For example, monkey B virus causes severe meningitis and infection of the brain. In my career, I have seen one case of lethal monkey B virus infection in a young student who was working with primates at a university research laboratory. This virus can be transmitted from a monkey bite; children have a higher risk of being bitten by a monkey than adults do, because children are more likely to unintentionally startle or aggravate a monkey. To protect both people and monkeys, I strongly discourage you from entertaining the thought of keeping a monkey as a pet.

Ferrets can spread many diseases to humans, including *Salmonella*, *Campylobacter*, *Cryptosporidium*, *Giardia*, and even rabies, influenza, and SARS, and have also caused severe injuries in children. For these reasons, they are not recommended as pets. The same is true for bats (yes, bats have been kept as pets!), which can spread many potentially lethal diseases, including rabies.

Horses and other animals that we typically associate with farms can also carry some infectious risks for people. I discuss possible infections from horses, cattle, and pigs in chapter 5.

Foaming at the Mouth: Rabies in Animals

When a child is bitten by an animal, many parents are concerned about rabies. Rabies is caused by a virus and is fatal if not recognized and managed promptly. In much of the world, including developing countries in Asia, Africa, and Central and South America, rabies is usually transmitted by dogs and cats. In these countries, rabid dogs are responsible for tens of thousands of human rabies deaths each year. In countries where most pets are immunized against rabies, including European countries, the United States, and Canada, the very few cases of human rabies are caused by wild carnivores, such as raccoons, bats, foxes, and skunks. Some European countries have managed to control and almost eradicate rabies in wild animals, and Florida has also had some success using baits to vaccinate wild animals, although such wildlife efforts can be expensive and difficult. In 2007, CDC declared that canine-strain rabies had been eliminated in the United States, but people and domestic pets still face risks from wildlife-strain rabies, as well as from the movement of infected animals across U.S. borders. Today, most rabies cases reported to CDC occur in wildlife, with bats and wild carnivores (raccoons, skunks, foxes, coyotes, jackals, and other species) serving as the principal hosts.

From 2000 to 2008, twenty-seven human cases of rabies were reported in the United States, and six of these people had been infected in other countries, including Mexico. Of the cases where infection occurred within the United States, most were associated with bat-variant rabies virus, even though many patients did not have a known bat bite. Despite a large focus on rabies in raccoons in the eastern United States, only one human death has been attributed to the raccoon-variant rabies virus.

At home, you can minimize the chances of rabies infection by having your pet dogs and cats vaccinated at regular intervals (every one to three years), not keeping wild animals as pets, and educating children to avoid contact with stray or wild animals, regardless of whether the animal is alive or dead.

If a child is bitten by a vaccinated animal, the risk of contracting rabies is minimal. In these cases, the animal should be watched for ten days for symptoms of rabies (aggressive and unusual behavior, extreme salivation, weakness, lethargy), and if these symptoms develop, the animal should be euthanized and its brain examined for the rabies virus. During the ten-day holding period, the person exposed to rabies should be treated at the first sign of rabies in the animal. The treatment should include both the vaccine and the rabies immune globulin. If, on the other hand, a child is bitten by a wild mammalian carnivore, a bat, or a domestic animal that is suspected to be infected, he should be immediately treated with the vaccine and immune globulin. If a child touches a dead or live bat or if you find a bat in his room (for example, in a country house where the window was open at night), seek medical advice right away, because cases of rabies in humans have occurred even without the person being bitten by the bat.

When traveling, you should be aware of the status of rabies in the country you are visiting. The world distribution of rabies is shown in map 1. In countries where no or few animals are vaccinated against rabies, every animal bite should be immediately and thoroughly washed with soap and water, because washing can prevent the virus from entering the nervous system. The bite should also be evaluated by a doctor, and in most cases, the rabies vaccination and immune globulin should be started. This

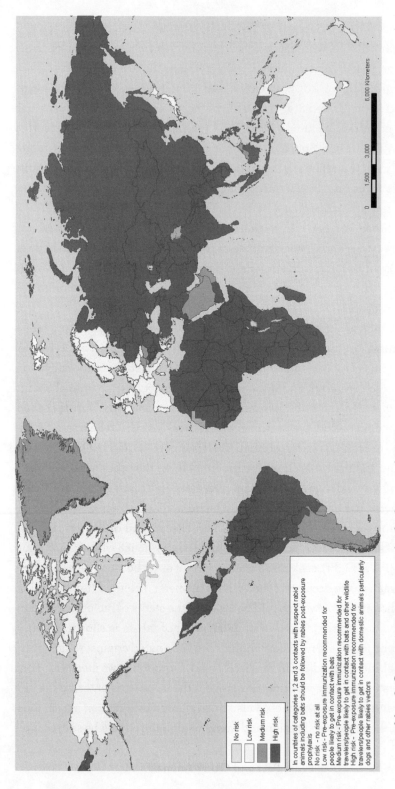

Map 1. Countries or areas at risk of rabies as of 2008.
Source: World Health Organization

In countries of categories 1,2 and 3 contacts with suspect rabid
animals including bats should be followed by rabies post-exposure
prophylaxis

No risk - no risk at all
Low risk - Pre-exposure immunization recommended for
people likely to get in contact with bats
Medium risk - Pre-exposure immunization recommended for
travelers/people likely to get in contact with bats and other wildlife
High risk - Pre-exposure immunization recommended for
travelers/people likely to get in contact with domestic animals particularly
dogs and other rabies vectors

No risk
Low risk
Medium risk
High risk

0   1,500   3,000   6,000 Kilometers

treatment can be stopped if the animal remains healthy ten days later, but frequently the animal escapes and cannot be observed.

Crossing the Species Barrier: Avian Influenza

I would be remiss not to mention avian influenza in a chapter about diseases spread by animals. Avian flu viruses occur naturally in wild birds and may not cause any symptoms in the birds that carry them or may cause generalized disease and even death. Usually, avian flu viruses infect only birds and not humans, a phenomenon referred to as the species barrier. These flu viruses are constantly mutating, however, so sometimes a subtype appears that can be transmitted from birds to humans, especially when people are living very close to birds. In Southeast Asia, many people keep chickens and other birds in or near their homes, and children even play with them as pets.

In 1997, an H5N1 subtype of the influenza A virus (of avian origin) appeared in eighteen people in Hong Kong, mostly children and young adults, and six of them died. Chickens and ducks were culled on a large scale to stop this outbreak. In 2004, the H5N1 virus reappeared in Southeast Asia, causing forty-six cases of flu in humans and thirty-two deaths. Again, most of the cases were in young people who had close contact with chickens in their homes or on farms. At the same time, outbreaks appeared in many Asian countries among chicken populations, and millions of infected and uninfected birds had to be destroyed. Migratory birds quickly transported the avian flu virus from Asian chickens to populations of wild birds in Europe, North America, and Africa.

To date, human cases of H5N1 flu have occurred in Asia, Africa, and the Middle East, but none have been reported in Europe or North America. As of July 2010, there had been 503 confirmed cases of avian influenza in humans, with 299 deaths (mortality rate of 60 percent). Currently, the H5N1 flu virus mainly infects people who are in close contact with infected birds. Transmission from human to human is still difficult, although it has occurred in a few cases with very close contact between a patient and a person caring for the patient. However, the risk remains that the virus may mutate further and become easily transmissible from person to person.

Scientists and physicians track the H5N1 virus, and intensive research efforts continue on developing a vaccine. At the moment, there is a pre-pandemic vaccine that gives partial protection to humans. Note that humans cannot contract avian flu by eating poultry. However, I recommend that children avoid close contact with chickens when they are playing.

MAIN POINTS
Measures to Avoid Infections from Animals

- Never leave young children alone with dogs, particularly large dogs.
- Teach children about safe behaviors around animals: Avoid unfamiliar, stray, and wild animals; never try to domesticate them. Do not touch dead animals. Do not play roughly with dogs or startle them while they are eating or sleeping.
- Vaccinate your dog and cat against rabies (including booster doses every one to three years) and vaccinate your dog against leptospirosis. Ask your veterinarian for the recommended vaccination program for these diseases.
- Have a new puppy (younger than 6 months old) medicated against worms before you bring it home, particularly if you have young children. Ask your veterinarian how frequently your dog and cat should be medicated against worms.
- Check your pet regularly for fleas and ticks.
- Do not feed your dog raw offal or a raw food diet.
- Do not let your dog defecate in playgrounds or any other place where children play.
- Remove dog feces from your yard at least once or twice a week. Never use dog or cat feces as compost.
- Teach your children not to kiss a pet or get their face too close to a pet's face and to wash their hands well after touching and playing with pets.
- Wear long rubber gloves to clean a fish aquarium. Wear a mask when cleaning a bird cage. Ideally, children should not do these duties.
- Avoid choosing a reptile as a pet and never have a wild animal or monkey as a pet.

5

The Great Outdoors

GERMS IN THE GARDEN, AT THE CAMPGROUND, ON THE FARM, AND AT THE BEACH

Whether out the back door or at a far-flung destination, the time children spend outside in natural environments offers valuable experiences and some of their best and most vivid memories. Most kids love to explore forests, beaches, and grassy meadows. While they are exploring, however, they may come into contact with a range of stinging and biting creatures: mosquitoes, flies, ticks, fleas, bees, wasps, spiders, scorpions, snakes, and jellyfish. Typically, animals sting or bite because a person is a possible threat or a possible source of food.

Contact with a biting or stinging animal may be short-lived, as with a mosquito, or prolonged, as with a tick. After a bite, saliva or intestinal contents from the animal usually get into the person's skin and may cause a reaction and sometimes transmit germs. Stinging animals do not transmit germs per se, but in many cases they inject venom, which can cause various reactions from mild to deadly.

In this chapter, I discuss the animals that children are most likely to encounter when they are outside as well as the consequences of a bite or sting. I also describe the best ways to prevent being bitten or stung, short of not going outside at all, which would not be much fun. Last, I briefly discuss some notable infection hazards when children are in the garden, camping, on a farm, and at the beach.

Bugs That Bug You: Mosquitoes, Ticks, and Flies

Bites and disease transmission by mosquitoes, ticks, and flies tend to occur during the summer in the United States, when insects are most abundant and people are more likely to be outdoors. Mosquito bites are particularly irritating; more than irritating, though, mosquitoes are vectors of many serious diseases worldwide.

Malaria is the prime example of a mosquito-borne disease that, every year, infects hundreds of millions of people and kills more than 1 million people. The risk of contracting malaria in the United States is remote, but because of its prevalence in countries where many Americans travel, I discuss it in detail in chapter 6. Mosquito bites in the United States, however, can transmit various brain infections (encephalitis).

Of all mosquito-borne diseases in the United States, West Nile virus is becoming most prevalent. The virus was first detected in 1999 in a few northeastern states; it then advanced to the south and west over the next several years and is now found in most regions of the country. Mosquitoes can become carriers of West Nile virus when they bite infected birds, and the mosquitoes can then pass the virus to humans.

Several thousands of people are infected every year, many of whom have no symptoms at all. About 20 percent of infected people develop symptoms, and some of these people die as a result. People of all ages are susceptible to contracting the virus, and older adults are most likely to develop severe illness. The symptoms include fever, headaches, body aches, and nausea. There is no specific treatment for West Nile virus, and mild symptoms usually resolve on their own. In the case of severe symptoms, you need to seek medical attention.

Some regions have mosquito-control programs, but the best way to protect children, and adults, from diseases transmitted by mosquitoes is to prevent being bitten. When you are outdoors in areas with mosquitoes, use an insect repellent that contains DEET. (See the box for a complete description of the safe use of insect repellents.) Wear appropriate protective clothing, including long-sleeved shirts and long pants, especially at dawn and dusk when mosquitoes are particularly active. Some outdoor clothing companies make hats, shirts, and other articles that incorporate

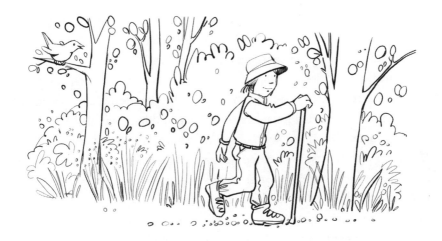

fine mesh in their designs so that the wearer is protected against insect bites without getting too hot.

In country houses and subtropical areas, install window screens to avoid being bitten indoors and have young children sleep under a mosquito net. In your yard, get rid of standing or stagnant water, which allows mosquitoes to breed, by regularly emptying water from plant containers, buckets, and barrels. Drill holes in tire swings to allow water to drain out, and change the water in birdbaths at least once a week.

Children are bitten by ticks more often than adults are, because children are more frequently in close contact with animals and their habitats. Ticks are usually found in dense, mature forests, in meadows with tall grasses, and in marshes. The main diseases that can be spread by ticks are borellia (Lyme disease), Rocky Mountain spotted fever, ehrlichiosis, tularemia, coxiella (Q fever), and hemorrhagic fevers. These relatively uncommon but potentially severe diseases are caused by germs that pass from an infected tick to humans or animals through a bite.

Lyme disease is the most common tick-borne infection in the United States. The disease is caused by a bacterium called *Borrelia burgdorferi* and is found mostly in the northeastern states, from southern Maine to northern Virginia. Some cases have also been reported from the upper Midwest, particularly Minnesota and Wisconsin, as well as from the West

Coast. The highest incidence of Lyme disease is among children between the ages of 5 and 9 as well as adults ages 45 to 54.

Typically, the disease causes a circular red rash at the site of the tick bite, but the rash doesn't appear until one to two weeks after the bite. Sometimes the rash is accompanied by flulike symptoms, such as headache, fatigue, fever, and muscle pains. Some children may develop meningitis or a usually temporary paralysis of the facial muscles (Bell's palsy). If children (or adults) are treated with antibiotics in the early stages, the disease will not progress. Later stages include a form of arthritis that usually affects the knees and other large joints, a type of meningitis, or involvement of the heart.

If you suspect that your child has been bitten by a tick, and she has a rash or other symptoms, contact your family doctor or pediatrician. Lyme disease is typically treated with antibiotics for two to three weeks, which gives a very good chance of full recovery, even though the symptoms (other than the rash, which clears up quickly) may last for several weeks beyond the course of antibiotics. Some experts recommend a single dose of the antibiotic doxycycline for children 12 years and older who have been bitten by and found an engorged deer tick on their body if they live in an area with a high incidence of Lyme disease, and especially if the suspected duration of tick attachment is seventy-two hours or longer. Contact your doctor if this situation applies to your child.

Another tick-borne disease, Rocky Mountain spotted fever (RMSF), is caused by the bacterium *Rickettsia rickettsi*. Humans can become infected from a bite by the American dog tick in the eastern and central United States and the Rocky Mountain wood tick in the western United States. Transmission of RMSF parallels the tick season in a particular geographic area, with the most common areas of occurrence being the southeastern and south-central states.

RMSF has symptoms of fever, headache, muscle aches, vomiting, diarrhea, and a rash. The rash usually first appears on the wrists and ankles and spreads within hours to the trunk, although it does not always develop, and it may be very difficult to see on black children. The illness can be severe and can cause meningitis, multiorgan failure, and death if untreated. Prophylactic antibiotics to prevent RMSF after a tick bite are not recommended.

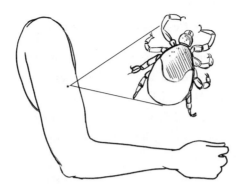

As for mosquito-borne diseases, the best strategy to prevent infection with tick-borne diseases is to avoid being bitten by a tick. When children are outdoors, they should wear appropriate clothing that covers their arms and legs. The ankle is a prime site for ticks and insects to bite, so if children plan to spend part of their day in the countryside or hiking in the woods, they should wear shoes that reach up to the ankle (boots or high sports shoes) and pant legs tucked inside their socks or shoes.

Insect repellents applied to the skin or clothing can also be effective against ticks. The safe use of insect repellents is described in the box in this chapter. When your child returns home, especially from an excursion to an area with woods or tall grasses, you should carefully check her whole body (including the scalp, behind the ears, and along the hairline) for ticks. Ticks usually cling to the skin for one to two hours before they attach themselves by embedding their mouthparts in the skin. The risk of disease transmission is directly related to how long the tick stays attached.

If you find a tick on the skin, you should remove it. First, grasp the tick with tweezers or gloved fingers as close to the skin as possible. Then apply even, steady pressure to pull the tick out straight. Do not twist it as you pull, because the tick's mouthparts can break off and remain in the skin. You also do not want to crush the tick or puncture it with a needle, because some of its germ-containing body fluids could enter the skin. Other methods, such as applying fingernail polish or isopropyl alcohol to the tick or holding a hot match to the tick, are not effective and can spread the tick's secretions into the skin. If pieces of the tick's mouthparts stay

What's the Best Way to Repel Biting Insects?

Several spray and lotion products are available commercially as insect and tick repellents. The most commonly used chemical ingredient in insect repellents is DEET (N-N-diethyl-M-toluamide). DEET is effective against mosquitoes, ticks, fleas, and flies when it is used correctly. Always carefully read about the content and strength of the insect repellent and the instructions for use on product labels.

The greater the concentration of DEET in the spray or lotion, the greater the duration of protection. For example, products containing 10 percent DEET protect for about two hours, and those containing 24 percent DEET for about five hours. Extended-action DEET products offer protection for six to twelve hours. The use of DEET has been studied extensively in children and has been found to be safe and effective. Nevertheless, always choose the lowest concentration that will be effective for the amount of time your children will spend outdoors, and apply DEET products on children's skin no more than once a day. In addition, don't use DEET products at concentrations higher than 30 percent on children, and don't use any DEET product on babies younger than two months, because a baby's thin skin absorbs chemicals more easily.

The best way to apply an insect repellent to a child is to put the

in the skin, trying to remove them can do more harm than leaving the small pieces there. When the tick has been removed, sanitize the skin with alcohol or another antiseptic. Preventive use of antibiotics is generally not recommended after tick bites.

If you have pets, keep them tick-free with the use of appropriate products. If your pet spends time in areas with ticks, such as marshes, forests, or cattle and sheep farms, you should carefully check its coat for ticks.

Flies can also be infectious disease carriers. The house fly, *Musca domestica*, can carry up to 4 million bacteria on its legs and body and up to 28 million in its stomach (yes, such studies have been done!). Flies are attracted by anything organic, including animal feces, so they are often abundant on farms and other places where houses are close to groups of repellent on your hands first and then rub it onto the child's skin. Keep the product away from open skin wounds or abrasions and avoid the eyes and mouth. When your children return home, rinse their skin well with soap and water or have them bathe to wash off the repellent. Combination products that include both DEET and sunscreen are not recommended for children (or adults). Rather, use separate DEET and sunscreen products, which can and should be used simultaneously.

Another active ingredient in some insect repellents is picaridin, which is also effective and can be used on children's skin. To be as effective as DEET, however, the product should contain at least 20 percent picaridin.

A third chemical used in repellents is permethrin, which is for use only on clothing and other articles. Never apply a permethrin-containing product directly onto the skin. This repellent kills ticks and insects on contact, so it can be useful to apply it on the outside of clothing, shoes, and camping gear. Follow the instructions on the product about how to safely apply it and how to launder items treated with permethrin.

A variety of "natural" insect repellents, such as citronella, are also available, but they are very ineffective compared with the corresponding chemical products. Citronella and other similar insect repellents should never be used as the sole means of insect protection in tropical regions, where malaria poses a risk.

animals. Whenever a fly lands on something, including food and water, it transfers some of the germs it carries onto that item. In this way, flies were the vectors for many outbreaks of typhoid fever, caused by a particular kind of *Salmonella*, at the beginning of the twentieth century.

Today, given improvements in overall levels of hygiene and regular waste removal, the chances of disease transmission from flies are lower. However, using a few simple prevention measures is always a good idea: keep trash containers well sealed, frequently remove pet feces from your house and yard, cover food on kitchen counters or picnic benches, install window screens, and keep a flywhisk or flyswatter handy.

Lice and fleas spread diseases extremely rarely, usually where living conditions are overcrowded and hygiene is poor.

Occasionally, a mosquito, tick, or other bite site gets infected, usually after a child scratches the bite. If the symptoms of redness, swelling, and pain get worse, rather than lessen, as the days go by, you should suspect an infection. The bite area may also develop yellowish secretions or pus, or the child may have a fever. In these cases, consult a doctor to find out whether an antibiotic should be prescribed.

Ouch, That Stings! Bees, Wasps, Ants, and Scorpions

Bees, wasps, and ants are all a type of insect called Hymenoptera. Many Hymenoptera species have a weak poison that can produce painful, but in most cases not serious, reactions after a sting. A bee, wasp, or ant sting usually causes pain or itching, swelling, and redness in the area of the sting; a reaction is more common in babies and small children. Applying ice or cold compresses on the area helps to lessen the pain and swelling. If part of the insect has remained in the skin, remove it by using a light hand. Do not press on the skin, because this may cause more of the poison to enter the wound. Older children can take antihistamines by mouth to help relieve the symptoms.

Although the vast majority of bee, wasp, and ant stings are not serious, about 1 to 4 percent of the population is hypersensitive to the poison of Hymenoptera. These people may develop an immediate anaphylactic (allergic) reaction. If someone develops symptoms of a general allergic reaction—hives, swelling (particularly around the mouth and on the face), or difficulty breathing—you should urgently seek medical help. People with a history of allergic reactions to Hymenoptera stings should always carry an epinephrine (adrenaline) injection, commonly called an epi-pen, especially if they are going to a remote location. These single-use injections are available in pharmacies and are easy to use. It is encouraging to know that four in five children who develop an allergic reaction to a bee or wasp sting will *not* have such a reaction after a future sting.

When camping or picnicking, you can minimize the chances of a bee or wasp sting by wearing a hat and light-colored clothing with long pant legs and long sleeves (insects tend to be attracted more to dark or brightly colored clothes). Also avoid wearing jewelry, perfumes, and scented cosmetics, all of which can attract insects. Cover food and be careful when drinking directly from soda cans, because bees, especially yellow jackets, often crawl inside open cans to feed. If a bee lands on your child, avoid slapping or brushing it away; bees do not usually sting unless provoked or frightened. Keep in mind that insect repellents protect against biting insects, not stinging insects.

Fire ants, originally imported from South America, are becoming a problem in the Gulf region of the United States. They owe their name to the intense burning sensation that follows their sting, usually within thirty minutes of the sting, along with an itchy, raised red wheal, or welt. Over the next twenty-four hours, the wheal usually evolves into a small pustule that can get infected if the child scratches it. Sometimes, a large local reaction or even a severe allergic reaction may follow a fire ant sting.

Fire ants are small and red or black, and they easily invade houses and other buildings. For prevention, avoid areas that fire ants inhabit and do not disturb their anthills. If your child is attacked by fire ants, brush them off immediately and apply ice or cool compresses on the stings to relieve the burning and itching. Antihistamines and corticosteroids may be needed for larger local reactions, and an epinephrine injection is the best treatment for a severe anaphylactic reaction—swelling of the lips, tongue, and throat; difficulty breathing; or collapse.

Scorpions live in many parts of the world, including in the United States, and have a fearsome reputation, but fortunately, lethal scorpion stings are rare. Most scorpion-sting victims have pain only in the area of the sting. A person who develops a generalized reaction to the poison will have symptoms such as agitation, fever, rapid heartbeat, sweating, vomiting, and low blood pressure. These symptoms usually appear within a few hours after a sting, and the person should get medical help. If an older child or adult is stung and symptoms do not appear within six hours, there is no cause for concern. Babies and young children are more vulnerable to the harmful effects of the poison and can develop seizures or even coma from a scorpion sting. Therefore, you should always seek immediate medical care for a baby or young child who has been stung by a scorpion.

Scorpions are nocturnal animals that do not attack humans unless they feel threatened. Prevent scorpion stings by being aware of their habitats; in particular, children should be taught not to put their hands between rocks, where scorpions hide. When camping or traveling in areas with scorpions, shake out shoes and clothing before you get dressed, and shake out bedding before you get in.

Eight Legs and Jaws: Spider Bites

Most people think of spiders when they picture a creature with eight legs, even though ticks and scorpions also have eight legs. Most spider bites in the United States result in no more than a temporary itch or rash at the location of the bite. Two species of spider can cause a severe reaction from their bite, however: the brown recluse spider and the black widow spider.

The brown recluse spider lives mainly in the south-central United States and in the Midwest, but it can be found in other areas, too. It is light or dark brown in color, small (between the size of a nickel and a quarter), and has a violin-shaped mark on its back. It prefers dark, secluded spaces such as closets, storage boxes, barns, garages, and other little-used areas. Shortly after a brown recluse bite, the person may experience itching, tingling, swelling, and redness. The center of the lesion may develop a dark color due to skin tissue dying (necrosis) and blebs, or blisters. Fever, chills, nausea, vomiting, and muscle aches may develop within twelve to twenty-four hours after the bite. Symptoms like muscle aches, abdominal pain, excessive sweating, or salivation indicate a serious reaction. In young children especially, a purplish or blanched lesion indicates a severe case of poisoning, and blood tests should be monitored carefully at the hospital.

Treatment of uncomplicated bites (when there are no generalized symptoms) by a brown recluse spider is to immobilize the affected limb, clean the wound, and administer the tetanus vaccine if necessary. The wound should also be covered and the patient given an antihistamine to prevent itching so that they do not scratch the bite area, which could lead to infection at the site. Always seek medical help if you suspect that your child has been bitten by a brown recluse spider.

The black widow spider may be found indoors or outdoors, usually close to the ground, such as under stones or in deserted rodent burrows. These spiders are indigenous to all parts of the United States. They are larger than the brown recluse, about the size of a quarter, and are shiny black with a red, orange, or yellow hourglass-shaped mark on the underside of the abdomen. The bite of a black widow spider causes pain within an hour of the bite, followed by burning, swelling, and inflammation at the site. Within two to three hours, symptoms such as weakness, dizziness, trembling, and abdominal muscle cramps may develop, and they can last for several days.

Anyone bitten by a black widow spider should be taken to the hospital, where the affected limb should be immobilized, and the patient should rest, taking pain medication and muscle relaxants as necessary. For very severe cases, an antivenin is available.

Help children avoid being bitten by a spider by teaching them about places where spiders live and by having them shake out shoes or other items where spiders may be hiding before putting a hand or foot in. Even young children can learn to recognize the markings and characteristics of the brown recluse and black widow spiders. Explain to them why they should tell an adult if they find one of these spiders in their home or play areas.

Rattle and Hiss: Snakebites

Many people are nervous about snakes and fear that their children will be bitten while playing outdoors. However, only about 200 of the world's 3,500 types of snakes are poisonous, not all poisonous snakes release their poison every time they bite, and the risk of dying, even after a poisonous bite, is less than 0.2 percent. About 45,000 snakebites are reported every year in the United States, and only about 10 deaths.

Most poisonous snakebites (95 percent) in the United States are by pit vipers, which live throughout the country, and the bites usually occur during the spring and summer months. Members of the pit viper family include rattlesnakes, copperheads, and cottonmouths. Vipers have a triangular head, elliptical eyes, a facial pit between the eyes and nose, and two poison fangs in the upper jaw. Nonpoisonous snakes have a more rounded head and eyes and they do not have fangs.

When a pit viper bites, its fangs make marks on the skin, and about 80 percent of the time, the snake releases its venom (envenomation). However, less than one-third of venomous bites lead to severe poisoning.

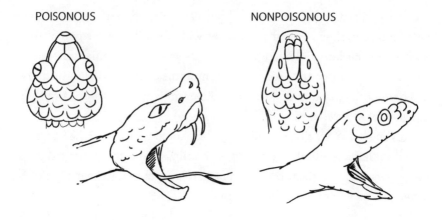

POISONOUS   NONPOISONOUS

A viper bite causes intense pain a few minutes after the bite, as well as swelling. The affected area turns a blue color, and in severe cases, the skin tissue dies (necrosis) and turns black. Some bite victims also experience general symptoms and signs of poisoning, such as rapid heartbeat, dizziness, fever, nausea, vomiting, neurotoxicity (weakness, tingling around the face), and low blood pressure (from which the person can collapse). Other victims may have symptoms of an allergic reaction, such as hives or difficulty breathing. Symptoms are often more serious in children than in adults, because children are smaller in size and therefore receive a higher dose of poison per pound of body weight.

Another native poisonous snake in the United States is the coral snake, found in Arizona, Texas, and the Southeast. Coral snakes are small, usually about three feet long, although they can be up to five feet, and have a small, rounded head. They are brightly colored with bands of black and red separated by narrower yellow bands. The rhyme "Red on yellow, kill a fellow; red on black, venom lack" serves to differentiate the coral snake from the similar-looking scarlet king snake, which is not poisonous.

Only about 40 percent of coral snakebites result in envenomation. The bite is only slightly painful, and other symptoms may not occur immediately. However, the lack of immediate symptoms should not be taken as an indication that there was no transfer of poison. In fact, serious envenomation is possible in these instances, and the bitten person should receive the antivenin before any symptoms appear. The coral snake's venom is neurotoxic, and symptoms can rapidly progress within a few hours from mild drowsiness to paralysis and death.

The first thing to do if your child is bitten by a snake is to determine what type of snake it was, if possible, and whether the snake released venom during the bite if it was a poisonous species. In the panic of the moment, it may not be possible to identify the snake, but try to get a good look at it and remember its shape and color.

If you know or suspect that the bite was from a poisonous snake or if the person is in intense pain, immobilize the area, apply gentle pressure on the extremity above the bite (between the bite and the heart) to restrict the return of venomous blood to the heart, and take the child immediately to medical care. Do not apply ice on the snakebite area, and do not try to suck the wound or open the skin with a knife, because you will only cause more damage to the tissues. At a hospital, the patient will receive supportive care with intravenous fluids, pain medication, antibiotics, and, if necessary, the antivenin specific to the type of snake. Ideally, the antivenin should be administered within four hours of the bite.

To minimize the chances of a snakebite, keep children away from areas known to be snake infested, protect their feet and legs by having them wear closed shoes or boots with long pants tucked into their socks or boots, and teach them to be careful where they put their feet and hands, particularly when disturbing rocks or piles of stones. When camping outdoors, shake out sleeping bags before sleeping in them at night, and check shoes and boots before putting them on. Explain to children that if they come upon a snake, they must not disturb it.

Out the Back Door: Possible Infections from the Garden

Many houses are surrounded by yards and gardens, where children spend time playing. A lot of children also like to help out with gardening work, which is a fantastic introduction to growing and caring for plants. Nevertheless, you should be aware of several infections that your children can contract from insects (discussed earlier in this chapter), animals, the soil, and even some plants.

As discussed in chapter 4, pets—yours or your neighbors'—and wild animals all frequent gardens and use them to urinate and defecate. Therefore, the soil can contain parasites such as *Toxocara*, which could then be swallowed by your dog or cat and later spread to your children. Because young children crawl or play on the ground and frequently put their hands in their mouths, they are more likely than adults to get sick from parasites on the ground and in soil.

Children who have a condition called pica, which causes them to eat dirt, are at particular risk of ingesting parasites, including one called *Baylisascaris*, which is excreted in the feces of raccoons in North America. Sometimes, children with pica become seriously ill from the parasites they eat.

Additional sources of infection in gardens are bacteria, fungi, and molds. For example, a stray cat that gives birth in or near your yard could transmit *Coxiella* bacteria, which causes a form of atypical pneumonia called Q fever (see the discussion for farms below). Birds' feces may contain fungi that can cause flulike symptoms; these are mostly of concern for people with a weak or suppressed immune system. Molds can become airborne and cause lung infections when moving old woodpiles, digging deep into the soil, or demolishing storage sheds or other structures.

Last, some plants can cause skin infections and other problems for people, usually through direct contact with the skin. For example, a rose bush thorn injury can cause the chronic skin infection sporotrichosis.

To avoid infections in the garden, have children wear long sleeves and pants and give them gloves to use when gardening. Young children should always be supervised while in a garden.

In the Wilderness: Possible Infections when Camping or Hiking

Many families enjoy camping and hiking trips. By spending long periods in the outdoors, campers and hikers are bound to come across at least a few germs that could lead to infection if they do not take precautions. Already described in this chapter are the flying creatures that can bite or sting, as well as animals like spiders, scorpions, and snakes. However, there are a few others to be cautious about, particularly those related to water.

It is important to stay hydrated when you are on the go in the wilderness, but it is not safe to drink water directly from lakes, rivers, creeks, or springs—not even when they are clear, cold trickles tumbling down seemingly pristine mountainsides. These waters can be contaminated with bacteria and parasites, such as *Giardia*, which can cause intestinal upset in humans. To ensure that fresh water is completely safe to drink, you have to either boil the water or filter and then chemically treat it with iodine or chlorine tablets at the recommended quantity for the recommended time. The filtration removes larger organisms (such as *Giardia* and *Cryptosporidium*), and the chemical treatment kills bacteria and viruses.

Giardia parasites are found worldwide and throughout the United States. They cause giardiasis, commonly called beaver fever, with symptoms of diarrhea, gas, abdominal cramps, and nausea. The symptoms typically begin one or two weeks after a person is exposed to the parasite and may continue for as long as six weeks. Dehydration is a concern with giardia infection, especially for young children, because they are susceptible to rapid dehydration when they lose fluids from diarrhea.

Swimming in rivers and lakes is a favorite activity for many campers. However, many wild animals, including rodents, also use these water bodies for drinking, feeding, and swimming, and they can contaminate the water with various germs. Infections you may be exposed to by swimming in lakes and rivers include

- skin infections from mycobacteria, *Vibrio*, *Aeromonas*, and *Pseudomonas*
- intestinal infections, such as *Salmonella*, *Shigella*, and *Campylobacter*
- other serious infections, including leptospirosis and *Legionella*
- meningoencephalitis (infection of the brain and its coverings) from an amoeba called *Naegleria fowleri*

In addition, when you swim in lakes or rivers, your skin can be penetrated by microscopic cercariae, a juvenile stage of the *Schistosoma* parasite. Most of the species of *Schistosoma* that affect humans are found in regions of Africa, Asia, the Middle East, and South America. Nonhuman (avian or mammalian) species of these parasites can be found in the United States, most frequently in lakes of the north-central states, but also in Florida and southern California. The U.S. species cause a red, itchy rash on the human skin that was exposed to contaminated water. The rash, also referred to as "swimmer's itch," can appear when the person is still in the water or immediately after she comes out, and it can evolve into blisters that may remain for up to two weeks. In other parts of the world, the *Schistosoma* species can cause more serious human disease that affects the internal organs, with symptoms that usually appear four to eight weeks later.

Another possible infection resulting from exposure to water is the outer ear infection known as swimmer's ear, which I described in more detail in chapter 3.

When swimming in lakes and rivers, avoid swallowing water and do not swim if you have open skin or mouth sores.

Horses, Cattle, and Pigs: Possible Infections on a Farm

Many of the infections discussed in both this chapter and chapter 4 can be encountered on a farm. Most infections acquired from horses are transmitted by ticks or mosquitoes that bite an infected horse and then bite a child. Some forms of encephalitis (infection of the brain) can be transmitted this way, including West Nile virus and eastern and western equine encephalitis virus infection, but overall, it is unusual to contract an infection from a horse.

Pigs can carry the bacterium *Yersinia*, which can cause gastroenteritis (and sometimes mimics the symptoms of appendicitis). *Yersinia* is transmitted through contact with pig feces or by eating food contaminated with pig feces (chitterlings are a well-recognized source of *Yersinia*). Also, as I discussed in chapter 1, eating undercooked pork can transmit *Trichinella*, a roundworm parasite that can cause gastroenteritis but can also progress to involve the heart, muscles, and lungs.

Another infection to be aware of is Q fever, caused by *Coxiella burnetii* bacteria. These bacteria are found in the urine and feces of infected sheep and cattle, as well as in the amniotic fluid and placenta of these animals. People are at higher risk of Q fever if they live on a farm where sick animals, animals that have just given birth, or animals destined to be consumed by the family are kept in the family's yard. Humans typically acquire the infection by inhaling the bacteria in fine particle aerosols generated from birthing fluids or by inhaling contaminated dust. Airborne particles carrying the pathogen can be spread downwind a half mile or more, contributing to sporadic cases for which there is no apparent animal contact. Unpasteurized dairy products can also contain *Coxiella*. People who live on a farm should keep sheep and cattle away from their yard.

Not everyone infected with *Coxiella* will develop symptoms, but those who do can experience acute fever, chills, headache, weakness, cough, and chest pain. Long-term symptoms can include weight loss, pneumonia, and liver problems. Rarely, Q fever can become a serious chronic condition, particularly in patients with underlying heart disease or prosthetic valves. Specific antibiotics can be used to treat Q fever.

There have been several outbreaks of infection from petting farms and zoos, with most of them involving intestinal germs. For example, a *Salmonella* outbreak in Colorado in 1996 was linked to a zoo exhibit of Komodo dragons. Although none of the infected children had touched the reptiles, most of them had touched the wooden fence surrounding the exhibit. Hand washing after a visit to a petting farm or zoo is the most important measure to prevent infection in your children.

Sand and Salt Water: Possible Infections at the Beach

Walking barefoot on a beach can be a great pleasure and is relatively harmless, unless you encounter a parasite. Parasites are present in the sand on many beaches around the world, especially in tropical and subtropical areas. One that causes a significant number of infections worldwide is the dog and cat hookworm, *Ancylostoma braziliense*, although several others may also cause disease. This parasite enters through the skin, especially when someone walks barefoot in contaminated sandy areas. Within a few hours, a rash develops and can form lines corresponding to the paths that the parasite has taken in the skin. The rash can be itchy—intensely itchy in some cases—and can last for months. It can be successfully treated by a single dose of a particular antiparasitic drug.

You can help to minimize the chances of infection by not letting your dog defecate on the beach.

Swimming in salt water, especially in the Gulf of Mexico, carries a risk of infection with *Vibrio* bacteria. People who work on boats can also be infected. These bacteria can cause wound infections through open sores exposed to contaminated water.

Jellyfish are common in many of the world's seas, including in U.S. coastal waters, although poisonous jellyfish are usually found in the South Pacific. A jellyfish sting causes immediate pain accompanied by a stinging sensation, and sometimes the affected area will swell and itch. Jellyfish stings in the United States usually end there with no further symptoms. In a few more severe cases, however, the person who has been stung may experience nausea, vomiting, headache, muscle aches, and, more rarely, seizures, coma, and shock. These symptoms develop anywhere from four minutes to six to eight hours after exposure.

If your child is stung by a jellyfish, rinse the area with seawater. Do not rinse with fresh water, because the cells of the jellyfish will break in fresh water, allowing more poison to be released into the wound. Apply vinegar to the sting area for thirty minutes or until the pain goes away. If vinegar is not available, rubbing alcohol or baking soda can help. Carefully remove any visible tentacles or other fragments of the jellyfish using tweezers and wearing two layers of gloves on your hands. Take your child to the doctor after a jellyfish sting if she has symptoms of an allergic reaction, such as hives, swelling on the face and lips, wheezing, or difficulty breathing. Corticosteroids and antihistamines might be necessary, as well as the tetanus vaccine, but antibiotics are not necessary. A doctor should examine the wound again a few days after the sting for signs of infection.

A skin injury inflicted by a sea urchin's spines can also become infected, though rarely. Some tropical seas in Southeast Asia have poisonous urchins. Last, in some parts of the world, although not in U.S. waters, there are sea snakes. Sea snakebites are usually very poisonous, and they constitute a medical emergency.

Prevent stings at the seaside by teaching your children not to touch jellyfish, Portuguese man-of-war (also called blue bottles), sponges, coral, or anemones in the sea or washed up on the beach. Jellyfish and other creatures can inflict serious stings for days after being on the shore. Stay out of the water if these animals are sighted.

MAIN POINTS
Measures to Avoid Infections while Outdoors

- Remove tall grasses and reeds from your yard, as well as all sources of standing or stagnant water.
- Use an insect repellent and follow the label instructions. Products containing DEET are safe and effective for use on the skin, but for use on children, they should not contain more than 30 percent DEET. Products containing permethrin are only for use on clothing and other articles, not directly on the skin. Do not apply insect repellent near the eyes or mouth or on areas of the skin with wounds or inflammation. When children return home, use soap and water to wash the areas where insect repellent had been applied.
- Avoid taking young children to areas where there may be a lot of ticks, such as wooded, marshy, and grassland areas.
- If your children spend time in an area with ticks, have them wear clothes that cover as much of the body as possible, including the hands and feet. Hats, long sleeves, and long pants with the legs of the pants tucked inside socks or boots are ideal. Devote a few minutes at the end of each day spent outdoors to checking your children's skin for ticks. Remember to check the scalp and hairline, the areas behind the ears, and the neck. If you find a tick, remove it.
- Keep your pet tick-free with the use of appropriate products, and regularly check its fur for ticks if your pet has been in a tick habitat or near agricultural areas.
- Make sure that children always wash their hands well after playing outdoors or with farm or pet animals.
- Explain to children why they should avoid drinking water from creeks, rivers, or mountain springs. It is also a good idea for children to avoid swimming in rivers or lakes if the water might be contaminated with animal germs.

- Seek medical care immediately after a child has been bitten by a scorpion or a snake. Monitor a child after a bee, wasp, or jellyfish sting, and if she shows any signs of an allergic reaction (swelling, hives, or difficulty breathing), seek medical care urgently.

Close to Home and Overseas

TIPS FOR AVOIDING GERMS WHEN YOU TRAVEL

The world is truly a smaller place today than it was fifty years ago. Transportation technologies have allowed travel to become a part of life for more and more people. For everyone, and especially children, travel offers educational experiences, an introduction to other cultures and lifestyles, and the opportunity to see and appreciate the world's natural wonders. In addition to recreational travel, many people travel for their work. Whether children are among the travelers or living in the home of a frequent traveler, they can be exposed to a variety of germs from other parts of the world. Even from a microbial point of view, the world has become very small.

In this chapter, I discuss the types of infections you and your children may be exposed to if you travel outside the United States, and especially to developing countries. Some of the illnesses I mention can be contracted when traveling closer to home, too, but on the whole, serious infections like malaria, dengue fever, cholera, and a few others have low or no incidence in the United States. I begin with some information about trip planning, including what type of medical kit to pack with you, and then I describe the main infections you could encounter. I also include a brief discussion of infections to be aware of if you are adopting a child from another country.

Getting Ready: Planning Your Trip

Planning a trip is exciting and can be a great way to involve your children in a family activity. There are so many things to think about—where to go, how to get there, where to stay, what to do, what to take—that it can sometimes be a little daunting as well as exciting. One particularly important aspect, and perhaps not the first to enter everyone's mind, is what measures to take so that you and your children stay healthy during your travels.

The risks of exposure to "exotic" germs, and thus appropriate health protection measures, depend on your destination, length of stay, and particular activities you plan to do. For example, will you stay primarily in Western-style hotels, spend time at a working farm, or be in tents on a wildlife safari? Staying in air-conditioned hotels carries a much lower risk of exposure to mosquitoes, which transmit malaria and other infectious diseases, than does sleeping in tents on safari. Some countries have a particularly high incidence of certain illnesses, so it may be necessary to have vaccinations before traveling or to take certain preventive medications.

It is wise to start inquiring about the possible measures you will have to consider at least two months before your trip, because vaccines do not take effect for several weeks after they are administered. You can ask for the necessary information for your trip destination at various places, including travel agencies, airlines, embassies and consulates, local health departments, travel clinics, and your doctor's office. Keep in mind that your pediatrician or family doctor may not have detailed information about exotic disease risks and the specific needs for immunizations for each country. For this, you should go either to a travel clinic, many of which are affiliated with a medical school or teaching hospital, or to an infectious diseases specialist. Do not expect your travel agent or others you deal with in planning your trip to automatically provide health information, and always check to ensure that the information you are given is current.

Reliable sources of up-to-date information are the Centers for Disease Control and Prevention (CDC, www.cdc.gov/travel) and the World Health Organization (WHO, www.who.int). Both organizations have search functions on their websites where you enter the name of a country and find specific recommendations about prevention measures, vaccines, medications, and other health and safety advice. Travel advisories are also listed.

Some of the infectious diseases you may be exposed to while traveling, especially in developing countries and tropical regions, are traveler's diarrhea, hepatitis A, typhoid fever, cholera, malaria, yellow fever, Japanese encephalitis, dengue fever, rabies, schistosomiasis, and meningococcal meningitis. Vaccines are available for some—but not all—of these diseases and are recommended for travelers going to certain countries. Prevention and symptoms for each of these illnesses are discussed later in this chapter.

Two other diseases, poliomyelitis and diphtheria, are also prevalent in many countries, but most people in the United States and other developed countries have been vaccinated as children. Nevertheless, a booster dose of the vaccines may be necessary prior to traveling. If you were not immunized against polio or diphtheria as a child, you can safely have the immunization series as an adult. A booster dose of the tetanus vaccine is also advisable in many cases, particularly if you plan an outdoor adventure trip.

Children in the United States should have received several vaccinations as part of their childhood immunizations. These vaccines include tetanus; diphtheria; pertussis; measles, mumps and rubella (the MMR vaccine); polio; hepatitis A; hepatitis B; chickenpox; hemophilus influenzae; and *Pneumococcus*. I discuss vaccines in more detail in chapter 9.

When you travel, even locally, and particularly when you travel with your children, I recommend that you take a first aid or medical kit with basic medications, sanitation items, and wound care items. Any medications should be kept in their original packaging to avoid possible problems during customs inspections. The kit's contents will depend on your destination, but in general, you should include:

- first aid items (gauze, cotton, Band-Aids, bandages)
- thermometer
- tweezers, small scissors
- sunscreen
- antiseptic wipes or gel
- cortisone cream for allergic skin reactions from insect bites
- antibiotic cream
- medications for pain relief (in liquid form for children)
- medications for diarrhea (*not* to be used for children)

- quinolone antibiotics for severe cases of traveler's diarrhea in adults (requires a doctor's prescription)
- electrolyte solution, such as Ricelyte or Pedialyte, to prevent dehydration in young children with vomiting or diarrhea
- chlorine pills or iodine tablets to make water safe to drink
- broad-spectrum antibiotics, if you travel to an area without good medical coverage (will require a prescription from your doctor)
- medications to prevent malaria (will also require a doctor's prescription)
- all medications that you normally take regularly

What to Eat? Food-Borne Infections when Traveling

Traveler's diarrhea, as implied by some of its many other names, such as turista, Montezuma's revenge, and Delhi belly, is a frequent and undesirable guest on many people's travels. In many parts of the developing world, tap water is not safe. Studies have shown that traveler's diarrhea affects about 50 percent of all travelers, and for those visiting places like India, Mexico, and African countries, this proportion is much higher. The local people are not as vulnerable because repeated exposure has given them some immunity to germs prevalent in their region.

In general, traveler's diarrhea is more frequent between October and May, particularly in Africa and South America, because of the rainy season that often causes floods and contamination of the water supply. Be wary even in places where you do not necessarily expect contaminated water. For example, in Saint Petersburg, Russia, periodic outbreaks of diarrhea have been caused by the parasite *Giardia lamblia* and other germs present in the city water. Also, the water from mountain creeks or rivers can appear crystal clear and pristine but still contain parasites, such as *Giardia*.

The most common germs to cause traveler's diarrhea are *E. coli* bacteria, and specifically enterotoxigenic *E. coli*, which are often abbreviated to ETEC. Other germs that cause diarrhea are *Salmonella* and *Shigella* bacteria and several parasites, such as *Cryptosporidium* and *Giardia*. People are most often infected by these germs when they drink contaminated water and eat raw fruits and vegetables that have been washed with contaminated water.

I discussed food-borne illnesses in detail in chapter 1, but I will repeat the main points here. Where there is any question about the water quality, you should avoid salads, fruits (unless you peel them yourself), tap water, and ice cubes. Remember the saying "Boil it, peel it, or forget it." Eat cooked foods right after they are cooked, when they are still hot, and be wary of milk and milk products that may not be pasteurized. Bottled water and drinks, as well as carbonated drinks, are the safest choices, even though they do not ensure 100 percent protection either, because their origin may not be reliable. In many developing countries, it is safest to use bottled water when brushing teeth, even in hotels, and to avoid swallowing water in the shower. The water in swimming pools can also have germs, particularly if the pool has not been decontaminated appropriately. In addition, chlorine, which is frequently used to sanitize pools, does not always kill germs like *Cryptosporidium*. See chapter 3 for information about safe swimming in a pool.

If you have the means, boil water to ensure that it is clean and safe to drink. Boil it for one minute after it reaches boiling point or three minutes if you are at an altitude greater than 6,500 feet (water boils at a lower temperature at higher altitudes, so the longer boiling time is necessary to ensure that germs are killed). Another method is to use filters (pore size of 0.2 microns) to remove germs, in combination with chemicals like iodine or chlorine tablets to kill germs. Iodine and chlorine are commercially available in tablets or in crystal form, and you add them to the filtered water in the recommended quantity for a specific length of time. Iodine should not be used for longer than one month and should not be used by pregnant women or patients with thyroid diseases. Also, as mentioned with respect to swimming pools, chlorination does not remove all germs, such as *Cryptosporidium*, for which filtering is recommended.

Children are more vulnerable to gastrointestinal infections, and when they get sick, they tend to have more serious illness, are at higher risk of dehydration from vomiting and diarrhea, and have fewer treatment options. The main treatment for traveler's diarrhea in children is to replace the lost water and electrolytes. Therefore, children should be given appropriate liquids and electrolyte solutions (for example, Pedialyte, Ricelyte) and a diet of boiled or pureed potatoes, bread, toast, rice, or banana, provided they are not vomiting. Children with traveler's diarrhea can also take antibiotics to speed up recovery; azithromycin is often a good choice. You should discuss this with your pediatrician prior to traveling.

Adults with traveler's diarrhea can take antiperistaltic medications to lessen the severity of the diarrhea, but these medications are not safe for children. In more serious cases of diarrhea in an adult, such as when there is fever or blood or mucous in the stool, a short course of antibiotics, such as quinolone, can be taken. Travelers should take these antibiotics with them from the United States and take them according to their doctor's instructions. Whether or not quinolone antibiotics are safe to use in children is still debated. Ideally, you will prevent traveler's diarrhea by being meticulous with food choices. With babies and very young children, the most appropriate option may be to avoid traveling to some destinations until children are older.

Hepatitis A is an illness caused by a virus and contracted by eating food contaminated by the hands of a sick person. Raw fruits and vegetables, water, and seafood are the foods that transmit hepatitis A most frequently. Foods from street vendors can also be risky and are best avoided, particularly by children. Countries with a moderate to high risk of infection with hepatitis A are shown in map 2.

There is a vaccine against hepatitis A, which is recommended for all children over 12 months of age in the United States. This vaccine has been licensed since the 1990s and was initially recommended in cases of international travel and in communities at high risk. In the United States, it was included in the general schedule of routine childhood immunizations in 2006. Therefore, if your child was born before 2006, he may not have received it. The vaccine consists of two doses given six months apart. Receiving only one dose is not as effective as having both doses, so advance planning is needed to ensure that you and your children are immunized before traveling. Having the full hepatitis A vaccine is the most effective way of protecting against this illness, which affects the liver and may cause symptoms of jaundice (yellow skin), abdominal pain, nausea, decreased appetite, and fever for a few weeks.

Typhoid fever is caused by a particular type of *Salmonella* bacteria which affects only humans and is found almost exclusively in developing

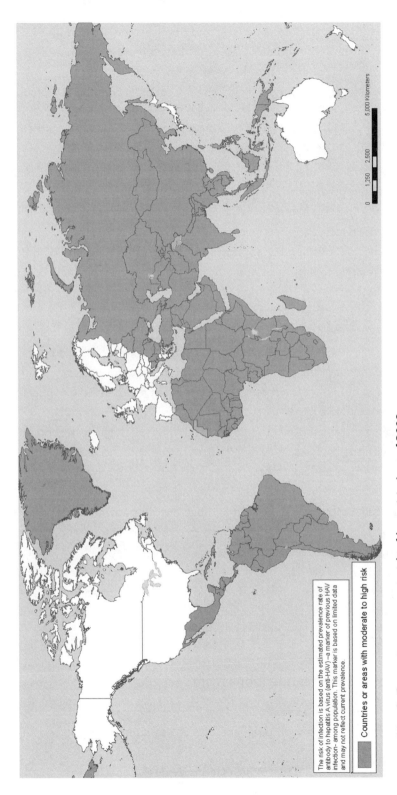

The risk of infection is based on the estimated prevalence rate of antibody to hepatitis A virus (anti-HAV)—a marker of previous HAV infection—among population. This marker is based on limited data and may not reflect current prevalence.

Countries or areas with moderate to high risk

0   1,250   2,500   5,000 Kilometers

Map 2. Countries or areas at risk of hepatitis A as of 2008.
Source: World Health Organization

countries (mainly in Southeast Asia and South America). The illness is transmitted through food and water that have been contaminated by a person who is sick or who has the germ in his stool.

Typhoid fever is prevented by avoiding potentially contaminated food, as described for traveler's diarrhea, and by a vaccine. The typhoid fever vaccine is available in several forms for different individuals, and the different forms offer varying degrees of protection (50 to 80 percent). Children from the ages of 2 to 6 years can have only the inactivated vaccine, which is given as an injection. From age 6 onward, children can also receive the live attenuated vaccine, which is given by mouth. The oral vaccine decreases the effectiveness of antimalarial medications, so ask your doctor about the most appropriate time to administer the typhoid vaccine relative to antimalarial medications for maximum effectiveness against both diseases. Neither typhoid fever vaccine is recommended for children younger than two years.

Typhoid fever is a serious disease, with symptoms such as general weakness, fever, chills, headache, muscle aches, lack of appetite, abdominal pain, and diarrhea. It can cause serious complications and even death. A doctor should always suspect typhoid fever in a patient who comes in with a fever after a trip to a country where this illness is common.

Cholera is transmitted through food and water that have been contaminated with the bacterium *Vibrio cholerae*, which is found in Asia, Africa, the Middle East, and South America, as well as (infrequently) in the southern United States around the Gulf of Mexico. Raw vegetables and fruits and inadequately cooked seafood and fish can all transmit cholera. The best way to prevent getting this illness is to be very careful about what you eat, as discussed earlier for traveler's diarrhea.

There is a cholera vaccine, but it is not very effective (only about 50 to 70 percent) and has adverse effects, so it is not recommended for travelers. Cholera causes severe diarrhea with loss of liquids and can be serious enough to cause death, particularly in young children.

Beware of Biters: Infections from Insect and Animal Bites

Malaria is a serious disease caused by *Plasmodium* parasites, which are transmitted to humans through the bite of the female *Anopheles* mosquito. This mosquito is most active during the evening, night, and early dawn hours. Malaria occurs in the tropical areas of Africa, Central and South America, and Southeast Asia, and also in some countries of the Middle East, as shown in map 3. It is a frequent disease in travelers who return from these malaria-endemic areas. Rarely, cases of "airport malaria" occur, which are believed to be due to the transport of mosquitoes on airplanes from endemic to non-endemic areas.

Several *Plasmodium* species cause malaria in different parts of the world, with *Plasmodium falciparum* in Africa being the most dangerous. In 2008, malaria affected close to 300 million people and caused about 1 million deaths. Many of the people infected and killed by malaria are children, because they are much more vulnerable than adults both to contracting the disease and to developing serious symptoms.

There is no vaccine for malaria, so the most important preventive measures are to take appropriate malaria medications and to avoid mosquito bites as much as possible. Preventive malaria medications (called *malaria prophylaxis*) are taken both before and during travel to a malaria-endemic country. These preventive medications are the most effective way to prevent contracting malaria, because completely avoiding mosquito bites is extremely difficult, and only one bite from one infected mosquito can transmit the parasite.

Before receiving malaria medications, your doctor will assess your health, because some of the medications require that you be checked for deficiency of an enzyme called G6PD. The medications may also differ for some members of your family, because some cannot be used in young children. In addition, your destination will play a role in which medication you receive, because the *Plasmodium* parasites in some parts of the world have developed resistance to particular antimalarial drugs. Depending on the drug, malaria medications should be started anywhere from one to two days to one to two weeks before your trip and should be continued for one to four weeks after your return.

With climate changes, the geographical distribution of malaria is changing, so you should check a reliable source, such as the CDC website (www.cdc.gov/malaria) for up-to-date information about the appropriate antimalarial medications for each part of the world.

In addition to taking appropriate malaria medications, travelers must

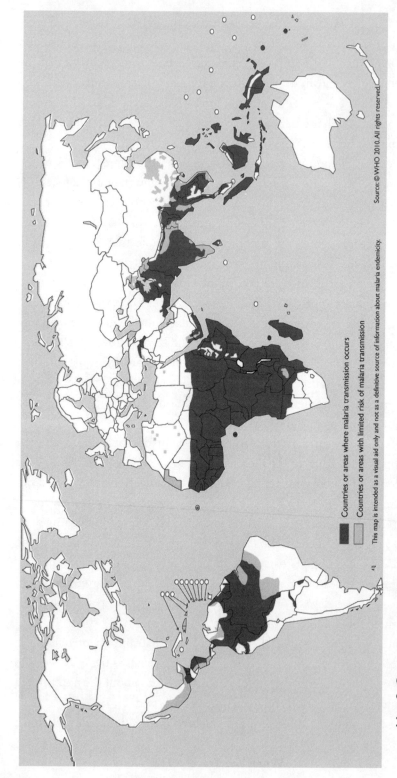

■ Countries or areas where malaria transmission occurs

▨ Countries or areas with limited risk of malaria transmission

This map is intended as a visual aid only and not as a definitive source of information about malaria endemicity.

Map 3. Countries or areas at risk of malaria transmission as of 2009.
Source: World Health Organization

do whatever they can to avoid being bitten by mosquitoes, particularly during the evening and night. Meticulously follow these three measures when you are in a malaria-endemic region:

1. Wear appropriate clothing, including long sleeves, long pants, and socks.
2. Use insect repellents on clothes (permethrin products) and on skin (DEET products).
3. Sleep under a mosquito net, particularly when in safari tents, and ideally, impregnate the nets with permethrin.

Recent research has shown that the chemical DEET (N-N-diethyl-M-toluamide) is safe and effective as an insect repellent and can be used even by young children in areas at high risk for malaria. DEET's possible side effects, including neurological ones, are extremely rare. The risks for children presented by malaria are far greater than the possible side effects of insect repellents. Nevertheless, DEET-containing products should not be used on babies younger than 2 months old and should be applied only very lightly around the eyes and mouth, even in older children. I discuss the safe use of insect repellents in more detail in chapter 5. Because the mosquitoes that transmit malaria are more likely to bite during the evening and night and into the early dawn, keep children inside air-conditioned buildings during these times when visiting malaria-endemic areas.

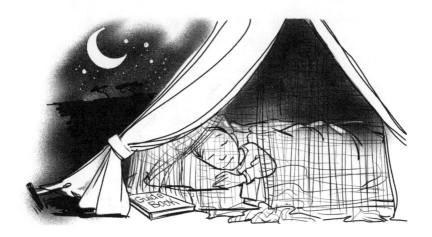

The symptoms of malaria are fever with chills that can appear periodically (every second or third day), headache, cough, abdominal pain, muscle pains, and, especially in children, vomiting and diarrhea. In children in particular, the disease can quickly cause complications in the kidneys, brain, and liver as the parasite destroys red blood cells.

Malaria during pregnancy is especially serious, with a high risk of complications for both mother and fetus. For these reasons, and because none of the antimalarial drugs is 100 percent effective in preventing the disease, pregnant women should avoid traveling to areas with malaria. If such travel is absolutely necessary, some (but not all) of the antimalarial drugs are safe and can be administered during pregnancy. It is also safe for pregnant and nursing mothers to use DEET.

Yellow fever is a viral disease transmitted to humans through mosquito bites in some African and South American countries near the equator, as shown in map 4; the disease is not found in Asia. There is a vaccine against yellow fever, which is recommended before traveling to endemic countries and must be administered ten days before traveling. The vaccine is given only in health departments and clinics approved by WHO. When you get the vaccine, you also receive a certificate of vaccination, valid for ten years, which you should present upon entry to a country with endemic yellow fever. The vaccination is not recommended for children younger than 9 months, pregnant women, or people allergic to eggs. These individuals should avoid traveling to areas endemic for yellow fever. The disease can cause mild flulike symptoms or serious damage to the liver, bleeding, and even death. There is no specific treatment for yellow fever.

Japanese encephalitis is a viral disease also transmitted through mosquito bites in several Southeast Asian countries, including India, Korea, Japan, and Indonesia. The risk of contracting Japanese encephalitis is low for travelers, especially those who are visiting an endemic country for a short time and who will be primarily in urban areas. The risk is higher for people who spend prolonged periods in rural and agricultural areas. A vaccine is available, but vaccination is not usually necessary for short-term travel (less than thirty days). Also, the vaccine should not be administered to babies younger than one year. The best prevention is to use insect repellents and avoid mosquito bites in the evening. Japanese encephalitis can cause a serious or even deadly infection of the brain.

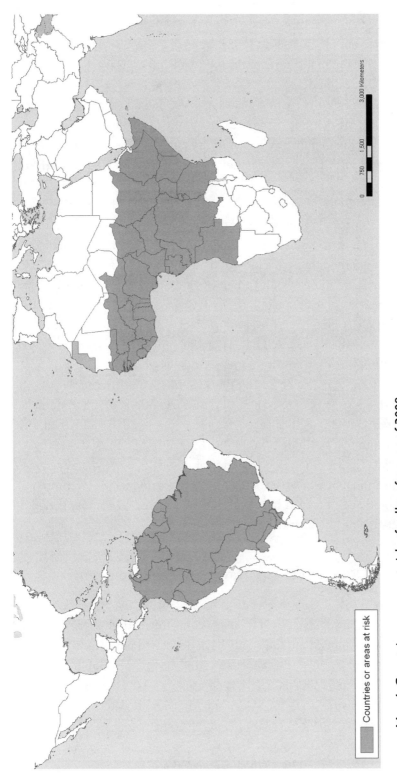

Map 4. Countries or areas at risk of yellow fever as of 2008.
Source: World Health Organization
Note: Yellow fever is not found in Southeast Asia.

Countries or areas at risk

Dengue fever is another viral disease that is transmitted through mosquito bites, but in this case, the mosquitoes are active during the day. Dengue exists in many parts of the world, including Hawaii and the Caribbean, Central and South America, and Asia. It has also become indigenous in Key West, Florida. There is no vaccine, so avoiding mosquito bites during the daytime is the best prevention. Dengue fever can cause a mild disease with flulike symptoms or more severe disease with intense muscle and joint pains, and sometimes fatal bleeding, particularly in babies.

Rabies is a viral disease that may be encountered by travelers who intend to stay for a longer period of time in parts of the developing world, particularly in rural areas or locations with many stray animals. The disease is transmitted through a bite from an infected animal, so you should avoid stray dogs, monkeys, and other wild animals. Exposure to the rabies virus is also a risk with spelunking, or cave exploring, particularly in the United States, where bat rabies is a problem.

There is a rabies vaccine, but it is not recommended for most travelers, because the risk of a traveler getting rabies is generally low. However, you may want to consider having the vaccine if you plan to travel to an area with a high risk of exposure to rabies from dogs or other animals, if you intend to stay in these areas for a long time, and particularly if you will travel to places where it might be difficult to find the vaccine if you do need it. The vaccine can be given to children. If you or your child sustains an animal bite in a part of the world where dog rabies is a problem, you should seek medical help and get the vaccine as recommended. I described rabies in more detail in chapter 4.

Other Infections Travelers May Encounter

Schistosomiasis is a disease caused by a parasite, *Schistosoma*, that is carried by freshwater snails. Humans become infected when they expose their skin to water where the snails have deposited parasites in tropical Africa, several Caribbean islands, and in some areas of South America and the Arabian Peninsula. There is no vaccine, so the best way to avoid this infection is not to swim, wade, or participate in water sports in any lake or river that may be contaminated.

Places that are definitely contaminated with *Schistosoma* include the Nile River in Egypt, all lakes in Africa (including lakes Victoria, Volta, Cariba, and Malawi), the Tigris and Euphrates rivers in Turkey, Syria, and Iraq, and many fresh water bodies in the Caribbean and South America. Swimming in chlorinated swimming pools and in the sea is safe from a *Schistosoma* point of view in these areas. Showering is also fine, provided the water has been warmed to over 122°F (50°C) for more than five minutes.

This illness can manifest several weeks after exposure to the parasite and can involve multiple organs with symptoms such as fever, weakness, cough, rash, abdominal pain, nausea, diarrhea, and enlargement of the liver, spleen, and lymph nodes.

Meningococcal meningitis, an infection of the tissues that cover the brain, is caused by the bacterium *Meningococcus*. The bacteria are transmitted from person to person by contaminated droplets from coughs and sneezes, as well as by close contact with an infected person. Meningitis mostly affects children and young adults. The *Meningococcus* bacteria occur throughout the world, including in the United States, but the so-called meningitis belt includes the regions with a higher frequency of the disease. These regions are near the equator in Africa (south of the Sahara), mainly in their dry season from December to June, and in parts of Asia and the Middle East. For example, several meningitis outbreaks have occurred during the Muslim pilgrimage to Mecca.

There is a vaccine against meningococcal meningitis, which travelers should have before traveling to areas where the disease is prevalent, especially during the dry season. It is also wise to avoid crowded areas, particularly with children. Meningitis has a high risk for complications such as deafness, mental retardation, and even death. I described this illness further in chapter 2.

Measles is a highly contagious illness that is rare among children in the United States, because most of them receive the vaccine as part of the recommended vaccination schedule. However, the risk of transmission is higher in certain countries, including some regions of Europe, Africa, the Middle East, and Asia. If a baby has to travel to a country with a high risk for measles, the measles vaccine, which is normally given after the age of 12 months, can be given earlier, between 6 to 12 months. (In this case, the baby must receive the measles vaccine again after the age of 12 months.)

Respiratory infections are common among travelers, because they can be spread easily in places where people are together for long periods, notably in airplanes, airports, and buses. Children are especially vulnerable. When my son was younger, he got sick with a viral infection every time he traveled on a long-distance flight. Airplane air has fewer germs than airport or bus air because it is recycled and filtered frequently, and it flows from the ceiling to the floor. Even so, several infections can be spread in an airplane, as well as on other transportation options, depending on how close a person's seat is to a sick individual's seat. Infections that can be transmitted include influenza, mumps, tuberculosis, and many others with respiratory transmission.

Influenza tends to be a seasonal illness, which means that during the Northern Hemisphere summer, when we get a break from the flu, it is present in the Southern Hemisphere. The flu is also present all year-round in tropical areas near the equator. A child older than 6 months should have the flu vaccine before traveling during the flu season (depending on the destination). As a general rule, I recommend that young babies (particularly babies younger than 3 months) not be taken on airplanes or other mass transportation to avoid exposing them to germs.

In addition to being exposed to germs en route to your destination, you may be exposed to germs once you get there, specifically at a hotel. A study in 2006 tracked adults who spent a night at a hotel while they had a common cold caused by a rhinovirus. The study found that one of every three objects these infected people touched became contaminated with a rhinovirus, and these viruses persisted for up to twenty-four hours on surfaces such as light switches, telephones, and remote controls. In many hotels, these objects are not likely to be cleaned every day, so pay attention to hygiene, especially of your children, when in a hotel.

Cruise ships are another place for viral infections to spread, typically noroviruses, which affect the gastrointestinal system. There have also been cases of people contracting pneumonia from *Legionella* in pools and Jacuzzis on cruise ships.

Last, but not least, travelers should avoid getting tattoos, body piercings, or acupuncture in countries where sanitation may not be a priority.

And although you may not have an option if you need urgent medical or dental care, it's better to leave medical and dental procedures until you return home to minimize the chance of contracting an infection from inadequately cleaned equipment or other unhygienic situations.

Growing Your Family: Adoptions from Other Countries

The number of children adopted from countries in Asia, Eastern Europe, South America, Africa, and the Middle East has increased markedly in recent years. Health services and medical screening tests are not necessarily as thorough or as available in many countries as they are in the United States. Therefore, you should have your adopted child checked for infections such as hepatitis B and C, HIV, and syphilis (which all require a blood test); tuberculosis (via a skin test and, if positive, a chest x-ray); and possibly lice.

Show your child's vaccination record to your pediatrician, keeping in mind that the records are not always reliable. For example, some doses of a vaccine may have been missed or a vaccine may have lost its effectiveness by being inappropriately stored. If in doubt about the accuracy of the vaccination records, special blood tests can show whether or not the child has immunity against the germs that cause vaccine-preventable diseases. A safe choice would be to repeat all vaccinations according to the schedule for children's vaccination in the United States.

⊢ MAIN POINTS ⊢
Measures to Prevent Tropical
and Other Travel-Related Infections

- Make sure your children have received all the recommended childhood vaccinations, including the vaccines against tetanus, diphtheria/pertussis, measles/mumps/rubella, polio, hepatitis B, chickenpox, hemophilus influenza, and *Pneumococcus*. Take your children's vaccination records with you when you travel, because some countries may ask to see them at customs. See chapter 9 for more information about childhood vaccination.

- Do your homework to find out what medications and additional vaccines are recommended for the destination you've chosen to travel to, and visit a travel clinic or an infectious diseases specialist (your pediatrician can recommend one in your area) at least two months before your trip. Depending on your destination, length of stay, type of planned activities, and your children's ages, additional vaccines may include those against *Meningococcus*, rabies, typhoid fever, yellow fever, hepatitis A, and influenza.
- Get the most recent information on health and prevention for the countries that you intend to visit at the CDC website: www.cdc.gov/travel.
- To avoid traveler's diarrhea, be meticulous about the food and water you give to your children. Remember the saying "Boil it, peel it, or forget it."
- Drink water only from reliable sources, which include reliable bottled water, boiled water, and filtered water treated with chlorine or iodine. Carbonated bottled drinks are safe. Avoid ice, unless you know it has been made from clean water.
- Avoid exposing children to mosquitoes in countries where malaria or dengue fever are endemic. Dress in long sleeves, long pants, and socks; use insect repellents (DEET); sleep under mosquito nets and, if possible, in rooms with window screens.
- If necessary for your destination, take malaria prophylaxis medications according to the instructions. Start taking them before your trip, take them during the trip, and continue to take them for as long as your doctor recommends after you return home.
- Consider carefully whether the destinations and activities you are planning are suitable for children, especially for babies and young children. Some more adventurous trips, like safaris, overnight tenting, and hiking, may be more appropriate for older children. The experience would certainly be much more fun and educational for older rather than younger children.

7

Sexually Transmitted Infections, Tattoos, and Piercings

HELPING TEENAGERS
NAVIGATE GERMS SAFELY

You may not like to admit it, but your "baby" is now a teenager. Adolescence brings many positive aspects, including physical and mental development and new abilities, as well as a few aspects that are not so pleasant for parents. Your teenager probably has a fierce sense of independence, a deficient sense of danger, and a handful of risky behaviors. The three topics included in this chapter—sexually transmitted infections (STIs), tattoos, and piercings—can cause infectious diseases ranging from mild to extremely serious.

Particularly worrisome for parents are statistics that show teens becoming sexually active at increasingly younger ages. In the United States, recent data show that 60 to 70 percent of high school seniors (aged 17 or 18) and 40 percent of ninth graders (aged 14 or 15) have already engaged in sexual activity. Moreover, 25 percent of U.S. adolescents become infected with a sexually transmitted disease before they finish high school. Clearly, it is never too early to begin educating school-aged children about sex.

Many teens also assert their independence by turning their bodies into canvases for tattoos and pincushions for piercings. These forms of body decoration are most popular among adolescents and young adults, with an estimated 13 to 23 percent of this age group in the United States having either a tattoo or a piercing (other than earrings).

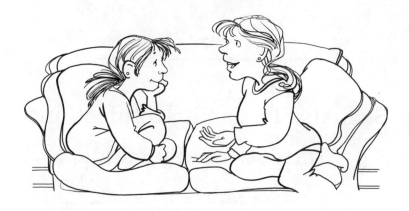

Not having sex and not getting tattoos or piercings are the only ways to prevent infections from these activities, but as parents, we all know our children will not necessarily take that advice. Therefore, what we can best do for our children is to make sure they understand the risks and know the precautions they should take. To give you the information you need to help your teen understand, this chapter discusses the infections that teenagers (and adults, of course) can contract from sexual activity and body decorations, including information on how to minimize the risks.

Of Concern: Sexually Transmitted Infections

STIs can be transmitted through many kinds of sexual behavior, including heterosexual and homosexual interactions, and vaginal, anal, and oral sex. The risk of transmission differs among STIs; some are easier to contract than others. In general, STIs are spread in one of two ways:

1. Through contact with a lesion or an open sore. Examples are syphilis, genital herpes, and human papilloma virus (HPV) infection.
2. Through infected urethral or vaginal secretions contacting mucosal surfaces such as the male urethra, the vagina, or the cervix. Examples are gonorrhea, chlamydia, HIV infection, and trichomoniasis.

The difference in how these infections are spread has consequences for how effective condoms are in preventing them, a subject I discuss later.

The risk of STI transmission during sexual activity increases with the use of drugs or alcoholic drinks because these substances impair a person's ability to recognize risks. Thus, it is less likely that a person under the influence of alcohol or drugs will take appropriate measures to decrease their risk of exposure to an STI. Studies in the United States have shown that one in four adolescents drank alcohol before sexual activity, and other studies found that college students who drank alcohol before sexual activity were less likely to use condoms and contraception.

Being infected with an STI such as gonorrhea, herpes, chlamydia, or syphilis increases the possibility of HIV transmission, in part because the first STI makes the genital organs more susceptible to HIV, and because the chances are greater that the person who transmitted the first STI also had HIV. In addition, most STIs are different from some other infections in that having a particular STI once does not provide immunity from the same STI in the future.

More adolescents and young adults have STIs than any other age group. One reason is the higher probability that they will have sex without using a condom, but in addition, young people are biologically more vulnerable to STIs. Moreover, adolescents and young adults do not always seek medical help, because they are embarrassed or scared, and often because they do not know the symptoms of STIs.

Protection against STIs

The most effective way for adolescents, and anyone for that matter, to prevent an STI is to avoid sexual activity. Teens and young adults need to know that their decision to be sexually active can have consequences for the rest of their lives. Sex can result in a pregnancy or in contracting an STI, sometimes both. It may seem obvious when stated so plainly, but it is a truth that many young people come to understand only after the fact.

Parents of teenagers know that teens often will not follow the advice to delay their sexual activity. As parents, we must teach our children how to protect themselves, just as we teach them all the other rules of personal hygiene. Safe-sex education should start early, in age-appropriate ways, because sexual initiation seems to be happening at a younger and younger age.

Short of abstinence, the best way to prevent transmission of an STI is the correct and consistent use of condoms. Condoms are not equally effective for all STIs, however. They are more effective for STIs that are transmitted through secretions (gonorrhea, chlamydia, HIV) than for STIs transmitted through ulcers, or open sores (syphilis, herpes) or HPV. Laboratory studies have shown that the germs that cause STIs, whether they are viruses, bacteria, or parasites, cannot get through the rubber of condoms. (Viruses can pass through condoms made of natural membranes, though, so these types of condom should be avoided.)

The fact that these STI germs cannot pass through a condom means that contaminated secretions from the penis can be contained inside the condom, and those of the vagina cannot infect a penis that is covered with a condom. However, STIs transmitted from contact with ulcers are rarely limited to the area covered by the condom. Therefore, although condoms can reduce the risk of transmitting an STI that causes an ulcer, they are not completely effective. A person with ulcers caused by an STI should not engage in sexual activity; unfortunately, as I describe in the next section, some people do not develop symptoms when infected by certain STIs, so they may be spreading the disease without knowing.

Latex condoms can be effective against STIs if they are used correctly, but what is the correct way to use them? To start with, condoms must be used every single time a person has sex, right from the very first time. Use only water-based lubricants, such as commercially available lubricants, because oil-based (petroleum-based) substances break down latex and make a condom less resistant. In other words, oils or lotions, such as Vaseline, applied on a condom reduce its effectiveness as a barrier and may allow some germs to pass through. Never reuse a condom.

Female condoms also protect against pregnancy and STIs, including HIV, but they are not as effective at protecting against STIs as male condoms; female condoms are thought to be 75 to 82 percent effective. They cover both internal and external genitalia and may be more cumbersome to use. They may be inserted up to eight hours before intercourse and can be used during menstruation or pregnancy. Female and male condoms must not be used at the same time, because friction can cause them to bunch up or tear. As with male condoms, do not use oil-based substances as a lubricant with female condoms, and use each condom only once.

Follow the instructions on condom packages about their correct use. In addition, adolescents should remember that other methods of contraception, such as contraceptive pills, do not protect against STIs, so dual protection methods should be used.

The only disadvantage from the use of condoms is the false sense of security that they may provide. They are *not* 100 percent effective. As you educate your adolescents about safer sex practices, be sure they understand that it is still possible to contract an STI when using a condom. Even though adolescents should be taught to use condoms "each time, from the first time," they need to know that only complete avoidance of sexual activity is 100 percent effective against STI transmission. Inform teens that consuming alcohol or drugs can impair their ability to make the right decisions and that they should limit the number of sexual partners they have. In addition, if you have a daughter, explain to her that she should avoid vaginal douching, because it alters the microbial content of the vagina, resulting in infections, and it can also push STIs farther up the genital system into the uterus and fallopian tubes. Finally, adolescents should know that STIs may not produce symptoms, but they can still cause complications to the infected person and can still be passed on to others through sexual activity.

STIs Transmitted Mainly through Contact with a Lesion

More than forty human papilloma viruses (HPVs) can be transmitted through sexual activity and can affect both females and males. Genital HPV is the most common STI in the United States, with almost half of all sexually active female adolescents becoming infected with an HPV. Some HPVs cause genital warts, which are also called *condylomas*, while others do not cause any symptoms. Years later, however, a woman infected by an HPV may have abnormal Pap tests and can develop cancer of the cervix. More rarely, HPVs cause other cancers, including, in women, cancers of the vulva, vagina, and anus, and in men, cancers of the penis and anus. Rarely, the newborn of an infected mother can get condylomas on the vocal cords, causing respiratory blockage. This illness can be very difficult to treat and frequently requires repeated surgeries. Although not completely effective, the correct use of condoms can prevent the transmission of HPVs to a great extent.

HPV infection can be very mild or may be without symptoms. Most infections are transient and clear up on their own. Warts may appear singly or in groups and can be flat, raised, or like cauliflower in appearance. There is no treatment for the viruses themselves, but anogenital warts can be removed with locally applied medications or with surgery. The warts may also go away on their own.

Today, there is a vaccine against some of the HPVs, which can prevent condylomas and cervical cancer. This vaccine provides a very high degree of protection and can be given to both girls and boys who are 9 years of age and older. Currently in the United States the recommended schedule is to give the vaccine to girls at age 11 and not as a routine vaccination for boys. This topic is a hot area of debate at the moment.

Genital herpes is caused by herpes simplex viruses, of which there are two types. The type 2 virus is the most frequent cause of genital herpes. This STI is transmitted by contact with the ulcers, or open sores, of an infected person. The ulcers are full of the virus and can easily spread the disease to the infected person's sexual partners. However, the ulcers can be so subtle that someone may not be aware of the infection and thus spreads the disease without even knowing it.

Once a person is infected with genital herpes, the virus stays in the body for life, although it will not always be active. The virus usually flares up at intervals, usually with stress as a trigger, and over time, the flare-ups tend to occur less frequently. Newborns who come into contact with herpes ulcers during birth can develop a very severe disease with a high chance of death or brain injury in those who survive. Some studies have shown a benefit from using condoms to prevent infection with genital herpes and others have not. On the whole, though, the evidence indicates a benefit.

Someone with symptoms of genital herpes usually has painful blisters that become ulcers in the genital area. There is no treatment to rid the body of this virus, but antiviral drugs can be used to treat serious symptoms or complications, frequent and severe flare-ups, and severe or generalized disease in patients with weakened immune systems.

Syphilis is caused by the bacterium *Treponema pallidum* and is transmitted through direct contact with a syphilis sore. These sores typically occur on the genital organs or in the vagina, anus, or rectum, but they can occur elsewhere too. Syphilis that goes untreated can result in a huge range of complications to organs throughout the body. In a pregnant woman, syphilis can cause fetal death, premature birth, or congenital problems (meaning problems or malformations present at birth). Some babies of infected mothers are born without symptoms, and years later, they develop problems with their brain, vision, bones, or teeth. In terms of protecting against the transmission of syphilis, as with genital herpes, some studies have shown that condoms work, and other studies that they do not. Overall, however, the evidence seems to indicate a benefit from using condoms to prevent transmission of syphilis.

In a teen or adult who contracts syphilis through sexual contact, the disease, if untreated, has three stages. It begins with a painless ulcer on the genital organs or other site of inoculation and then progresses within a month or two to the lymph nodes, causing a whole-body illness with fever, muscle aches, and a rash, even on the palms of the hands and soles of the feet. The symptoms of syphilis in the first two stages will eventually resolve on their own, but an untreated person remains infected. At the third stage, which may not begin for years after the initial infection, the heart or other major organs become damaged, and the illness may cause paralysis, blindness, or dementia. The brain can be affected at any stage of syphilis. Syphilis can be treated with antibiotics at any stage, but organ damage is permanent.

STIs Transmitted Mainly through Secretions

The bacterium *Chlamydia trachomatis* causes an STI that commonly occurs together with gonorrhea (discussed next) in the same person. Chlamydia is transmitted through genital and rectal secretions and is very frequent in teenagers, who are more susceptible to the infection than older individuals. Chlamydia is sometimes called a "silent" disease, because many infected people do not develop any symptoms. Yet, even without symptoms, the disease may cause significant damage for females by infecting and permanently damaging the fallopian tubes, uterus, and other tissues in the reproductive tract. The result can be infertility, ectopic pregnancy (pregnancy outside the uterus, a life-threatening situation), and pelvic pain. Males with untreated chlamydia infection are less likely to develop complications, although the epididymis can become infected (epididymitis). During birth from an infected mother, a newborn can develop eye and lung infections. When used correctly, condoms prevent the transmission of chlamydia.

When they do occur, symptoms of chlamydia are similar to those of gonorrhea, including abnormal discharge from the vagina or the urethra in the male and a burning feeling while urinating. A person without symptoms can still spread the infection to sexual partners. Chlamydia is easily treatable with antibiotics. Annual chlamydia testing is recommended for sexually active females younger than 25 years of age.

Gonorrhea, caused by the bacterium *Neisseria gonorrhoeae*, is also transmitted through secretions from the genital or rectal mucosal membranes. Rarely, it can be spread through contaminated objects such as bed sheets. Adolescent girls are at greater risk than older women for contracting gonorrhea. For females, the danger from gonorrhea is that it can cause severe inflammation in the pelvis, and the inflammation can extend to the uterus and fallopian tubes, resulting in future fertility problems. For males, gonorrhea can cause epididymitis and fertility problems. Babies born vaginally from an infected mother can develop an eye infection. When used correctly, condoms prevent the transmission of gonorrhea.

The symptoms of gonorrhea are a discharge that looks like pus coming from the vagina or, in males, the urethra, and pain during urination. These symptoms are often very mild or even nonexistent. A person without symptoms can still spread gonorrhea, however, through sexual contact to a partner. Gonorrhea can be treated with antibiotics, although the infection is becoming more difficult to treat because the germ has developed resistance to some antibiotics.

Trichomoniasis is a common STI caused by a parasite called *Trichomonas vaginalis*. Both females and males can be infected with this parasite, which can cause some unpleasant symptoms but generally does not cause health complications. When used correctly, condoms prevent the transmission of *Trichomonas*. Typical symptoms in females are a vaginal discharge and a burning or itching sensation in the vagina. Males usually do not have symptoms, although some men experience pain or burning when they urinate. Trichomoniasis can be treated with antibiotics.

Hepatitis B and C infections are caused by viruses that can be spread through secretions, including semen and vaginal fluids, and blood. In both females and males, these viruses can cause acute or chronic inflammation of the liver (hepatitis), and the disease can lead to liver failure or cancer. The transmission of hepatitis B and C viruses may be prevented by condoms, but no studies have shown this conclusively. There is no satisfactory treatment for these infections, although many promising new drugs are in development. A vaccine against hepatitis B is available and is recommended for all children. A baby born to a woman with hepatitis B should receive one dose of the vaccine within the first twelve to twenty-four hours of life, along with the specific immune globulin. Two more doses of the vaccine are necessary during the baby's first six months.

The human immunodeficiency virus (HIV) causes the most severe STI, because, to date, there is no radical cure for the virus or for the disease it leads to, acquired immune deficiency syndrome (AIDS). About half of all new cases of HIV each year in the United States occur in adolescents and young adults. HIV is one of the main causes of death in people between the ages of 15 and 24 years. The primary route of infection in this age group is sexual activity, specifically transmission from semen and vaginal secretions, but the virus can also be contracted by using contaminated needles, by the blood of an infected person coming in contact with the mucosal membranes or injured skin of an uninfected person, and by a baby of an infected mother during pregnancy, delivery, or breastfeeding.

The virus attacks the immune system, and the resulting immune suppression makes an infected person particularly vulnerable to various other infections caused by bacteria, viruses, parasites, and fungi, which can affect any part of the body. Compared with other STIs, HIV is not very contagious, but do not let this fact mislead you. Despite HIV being less contagious than other STIs, it is a serious and, at the moment, lifelong infection. Studies have shown that, short of abstinence, the best way to protect against HIV infection is the correct and consistent use of condoms.

HIV does not cause visible symptoms on the genital organs. Sometimes, soon after infection, a person experiences flulike symptoms, with fever, lymph node enlargement, muscle aches, weakness, and rash. Oftentimes, however, there are no symptoms. The virus can remain "silent" for many months or even years, but progressively it leads to symptoms such as lymph node enlargement, weight loss, diarrhea, neurological disorders, and an array of opportunistic infections.

HIV infection, which first appeared in the 1980s, has caused a large wave of research activity, and as a result, there has been great progress both in treating HIV infection and AIDS and in treating other AIDS-related opportunistic infections. Today there is long-term, lifelong therapy with combinations of antiviral drugs, so AIDS is not the death sentence it used to be twenty years ago.

If Your Child Is Exposed to an STI

If you or your child is concerned about possible exposure to an STI, you should seek medical help immediately. Even without symptoms, it is better to check than worry. Any symptoms like pain, unusual discharge, rash, ulcer, or other lesions on the genitals require evaluation by a doctor. A doctor can evaluate your child by conducting a physical examination and by taking blood, urine, and genital fluid samples for laboratory tests. If an HIV or hepatitis B test returns a negative result (meaning that the child did not test positive for the infection), the test should be repeated at least three to six months later, because it can take time for these infections to be detected in the blood.

STIs are common and often asymptomatic in young people. For this reason, as well as the facts that treatment options are available for most STIs and that treatment is better started as soon as possible, every sexually active young person should be checked once or twice a year for STIs.

Blood Transfusions

Many infectious agents can be carried in an infected person's blood, so blood transfusions needed in the cases of severe injury, surgery, and some diseases could be a possible source of infection. In the past, there have been such cases, but in developed countries today, transfusions have become very safe. They may not always be safe in some countries where resources are limited, however.

In the United States and other developed countries, donated blood is checked for HIV, hepatitis B and C, syphilis, HTLV 1 and 2 (which are viruses that cause a rare form of leukemia and neurological disease), and, in some cases, cytomegalovirus (which is one of the herpes viruses). The risk of germ transmission after a transfusion is not zero, but it is extremely small.

Body Art: Tattoos and Piercings

Tattoos and body piercings have been done for thousands of years in many cultures around the world. In the United States and other Western cultures, the popularity of tattoos and piercings on various parts of the body has increased. As a result, the methods used to apply tattoos and make piercings have improved and been standardized so that they are safer for both the client and the technician. Unfortunately, however, many tattoos and piercings continue to be done without using correct antiseptic procedures.

Adolescents should not attempt to do tattoos or piercings themselves. Also, people with preexisting conditions that increase the risk of complications from infections should avoid getting tattoos or piercings. Preexisting conditions of concern include congenital heart disease (a heart condition present at birth), disease of the heart valves, and severe skin conditions, as well as disorders that weaken the immune system. A person with one of these conditions has a higher risk of endocarditis, which is a serious infection of the heart, and of sepsis, which is a severe whole-body infection.

Tattoos

The tools for tattooing have changed, but the basic technique remains the same: a pigment or ink is applied at a depth of 1 to 2 mm in the skin using various devices. In the past, common devices were knives and other pointed objects, but now electrical devices can achieve the same effect with more control and less pain. Tattoo inks can be derived from ashes, oils, or synthetic dyes.

Whenever the skin—an incredible natural barrier for the body—is wounded, there is a risk of infection. Infections during tattooing can be caused by the germs normally found on the skin of the person receiving the tattoo. For example, *Staphylococcus* and *Streptococcus* bacteria can be part of the normal set of microbes that live on a person's skin. On the outside of the skin, they usually do no harm, but once they get through the skin barrier, they can produce local inflammation or an abscess. Less commonly, these bacteria can cause a severe whole-body infection.

Infections from tattooing can also be caused by other germs, ones that are not initially on the person receiving the tattoo. For example, in the last fifty years, many cases of hepatitis have been reported after tattoos. In some cases, the tattoo technician had recently been ill with jaundice and hepatitis and checked the needle on him or herself first before using it on the client. In other cases, the technician used needles that had been contaminated by use on other clients or needles or dye that had not been properly sterilized. HIV infection has also been reported in at least one person after a tattoo; this case was in a prisoner who used a needle previously used by others. Tuberculosis and even syphilis have been reported when infected people mixed their saliva with the tattoo dye.

Contracting any of these infections from getting a tattoo should be extremely rare, provided that the technician uses strict antiseptic techniques. Some states regulate tattoo technicians, requiring them to take health and safety courses and to be licensed. Regardless of licensing requirements, tattoo technicians should use the following antiseptic techniques. Ask your technician whether he or she does, and be alert during the tattooing.

- Clean the skin where the tattoo is to be placed with an antiseptic solution before tattooing begins.
- Properly sterilize tools between each client.
- Use single-use tubes of tattoo ink that are discarded between clients.
- Wear disposable gloves.
- Disinfect tabletops and other such equipment after each client.

In addition, the person receiving the tattoo should be immunized against tetanus. As the skin is pierced during the tattooing process, there is usually a small amount of bleeding, so new tattoos should be covered with a bandage until the bleeding stops completely. Essentially, a new tattoo should be treated as a skin wound.

Piercings

In Western cultures, earlobe piercing is common, with 80 to 90 percent of women in the United States having at least one pair of earrings. An increasing number of men also have earrings. Recently, piercings in the nose, lips, eyebrow, tongue, nipples, navel, genitals, and other parts of the body have become much more frequent. After the ear lobes, the navel is the next most common location for piercings.

As a pediatrician, I have seen several cases of earlobe infection in young girls, as well as cases in which the entire earring entered the earlobe. (In this situation, the earring should be removed with an incision on the lobe and not re-inserted for months, at least. Antibiotics are also needed.) I do not recommend earlobe piercings in young children. Rather, I suggest that you let your child make the decision for herself at an older age.

The risk of infection from a piercing depends on the part of the body being pierced, the technique used, the experience of the person who inserts the jewelry, and the quality of the subsequent wound care. Piercing technicians mainly use one of two techniques to pierce a body part and insert jewelry. One technique uses a sharp needle made of stainless steel to insert the open end of the jewelry through the skin, and the other uses an automated "gun" that pushes the jewelry through under pressure.

As with tattoos, infections can originate from germs on the skin of the person receiving the piercing or from external germs. Infections are most common in the navel, where piercings sometimes take months to heal, followed by the ears, nose, and nipples. Piercings on the tongue, genitals, and other parts of the body become infected less often.

Ears are usually pierced with an automated piercing gun, but these tools are difficult to thoroughly disinfect, although a new type of piercing gun is now available with a sterile disposable cartridge. The cartridge completely encloses the earring and is the only part that comes in contact with the customer. Local infections of the ear lobe are usually caused by *Staphylococcus* or *Streptococcus* bacteria, and infections of the cartilage of the ear (an increasingly popular place for ear piercings) are usually caused by the germ *Pseudomonas*. Cartilage has a smaller blood supply than the ear lobe and therefore has a greater risk of bacterial infection. In rare cases, an infection can spread from the ear to the rest of the body and cause complications in the kidneys or heart.

Infections from piercings in the navel and the nose are usually caused by the bacterium *Staphylococcus*. In the genital area, piercings have flared up HPV infections with recurrent warts occurring at the site of piercing. A range of infections have been reported from tongue piercings, including infection of the tongue (glossitis), abscesses in the throat, and infections extending to the neck or even the heart or brain, as well as generalized infections. Germs found in the mouth can be implicated in these infections, as well as staph bacteria and even HPV.

Hepatitis B or C can also be transmitted during piercing of any body part if the technique is not aseptic, such as when contaminated tools are reused. Infection with HIV has not been reported but remains a possibility. To prevent infection from piercings, the location to be pierced should be cleaned with an antiseptic solution just prior to piercing, needles should be used only once, all tools that are reused should be appropriately sterilized, and automatic piercing guns that don't have single-use cartridges should be avoided for ear piercing.

The time needed for a piercing wound to heal depends on the blood supply to the area and the condition of the tissues (for example, the tissues may have been injured if multiple attempts were made during the piercing). While a piercing heals, it should be treated with regular wound care. Professional technicians should provide appropriate aftercare instructions, which depend on the site of piercing. For genital piercings, sexual activity should be avoided until the site heals. The Association of Professional Piercers provides general aftercare recommendations on its website (www.safepiercing.org). If signs of infection develop, including redness, swelling, increasing pain in the days following the piercing, or fever, your child should see a doctor.

In addition to infections, some people experience allergic reactions to the metal of the jewelry, which is usually steel, titanium, gold, or acrylic. Nickel is not recommended due to the risk of local allergic reactions.

Measures to Help Adolescents Avoid STIs and Infections from Tattoos and Piercings

- Educate your adolescents about the reasons to delay sexual activity until they are adults.
- Educate your adolescents about how sex can be safer: use condoms correctly and consistently every time from the first time, avoid drugs and alcohol, and limit the number of partners.
- Avoid having young children's ears pierced.
- Explain to your children the infection risks from tattoos and body piercings.
- If your adolescent insists on a tattoo or a piercing, be sure she chooses a professional technician who uses aseptic techniques, sterile tools, and single-use needles.
- People with congenital heart disease, disease of the heart valves, severe skin conditions (such as severe eczema), or weakened immunity should avoid tattoos and piercings.
- Vaccinate boys and girls against hepatitis B and girls (only, for the time being) against human papilloma viruses.

PART II

Our Defenses
against Germs

8

Taking Medicine

THE USE AND MISUSE OF ANTIBIOTICS

Both as a mother and as a pediatrician, I know how much parents worry when their child gets sick. Even minor and common childhood illnesses, like colds, coughs, diarrhea, and earaches, cause a huge amount of anxiety for mothers and fathers alike. All that parents want is for their child to get better as soon as possible.

Parents often take a sick child to the doctor for treatment. For many people, proper treatment equals antibiotics, and they may be surprised, or even disappointed, when the doctor tells them that their child does not need antibiotics. After all, haven't antibiotics saved millions of lives and defeated so many infectious diseases? Surely, then, the reasoning goes, antibiotics should be used to treat all infections, even mild ones. But no, that is not what should be done.

Over the last several years, it has become increasingly obvious that the inappropriate and excessive use of antibiotics has many hazards, both for the patient who takes the antibiotics and for the wider community. One hazard is that antibiotics have side effects. A second hazard is that germs can—and do—develop resistance to antibiotics, rendering many previously effective antibiotics essentially useless today. If your child takes an antibiotic that she does not really need, this puts her at risk both while she is taking the antibiotic and in the future. In this chapter, I discuss these risks, as well as describe what antibiotics are, where they come from, and how they should and should not be used.

What Are Antibiotics?

In Greek, the word *bios* means life, so an antibiotic is a substance that acts against living organisms, in this case against microorganisms. An antibiotic can also be called an antimicrobial. The term antibiotic is actually used in a confusing way; it is used as a synonym to antibacterials, or substances that act against bacteria. However, there are also antimicrobials against viruses (antivirals), fungi like yeast and molds (antifungals), and parasites (antiparasitics). Most of the antimicrobials available for medical purposes are antibacterial. To avoid confusion for the remainder of this chapter, and in fact throughout this book, I use the term antibiotic to mean antibacterial. When I refer to other antimicrobials, I call them antivirals, antifungals, or antiparasitics.

The first antibiotics were themselves products of live microorganisms, but today most antibiotics are chemically synthesized. Some antibiotics are *wide spectrum*, meaning they act against many types of bacteria. Others are narrow spectrum, acting against only a few types of bacteria. Antibiotics work by damaging or killing bacteria, and they can do so generally without attacking the cells in a person's body because of fundamental differences between animal cells and bacterial cells.

Some antibiotics, such as penicillin and cephalosporins, kill bacteria by, for example, punching holes in their cell wall or preventing them from making their cell wall. Other antibiotics, such as tetracyclines and erythromycin, work by suppressing the bacterial cells' ability to reproduce themselves; for example, the antibiotic may shut down the machinery that makes proteins.

Everyone has billions of microorganisms living on their skin, in their intestines, and in their mouth, and most of these organisms do not cause disease. Indeed, some of them play an important role in health; for example, some microbes help us digest food, and others produce substances like vitamin K to make blood coagulate. When a person takes an antibiotic for an infection, the antibiotic will kill not only the pathogenic, or disease-causing, microbes causing the infection but also many of the harmless and beneficial microorganisms in the body. Destroying the good microbes can disrupt the microbial balance in the body's "ecosystem." Sometimes, fungi may take the place of the good microbes in mu-

Penicillin: The First Antibiotic

Antibiotics are one of the most important medical discoveries of the twentieth century. The first antibiotic, penicillin, was discovered almost by chance. In 1928, the British scientist Alexander Fleming returned to his laboratory after a few days' absence and saw some Petri dishes with microbial cultures that had been left in the sink. A fungus had grown in the dishes and was inhibiting the growth of a common bacterium, *Staphylococcus*. Fleming thought that the fungus must be producing a substance with antibacterial action. The fungus was a type of *Penicillium*, so he called the antibacterial substance penicillin. Although Fleming is credited with this discovery and with creating the term *antibiotic*, his experiments did not succeed in isolating penicillin.

A decade later, two other researchers in England, Howard Florey and Ernst Chain, restarted the experiments and succeeded in extracting penicillin. Other researchers in Europe and North America managed to produce enough penicillin to start clinical studies in animals and later in humans. In 1941, it was shown that even small amounts of penicillin could cure very serious infections and save many human lives. Fleming, Florey, and Chain won the Nobel Prize for Medicine and Physiology in 1945 for the discovery of penicillin.

Pharmaceutical companies soon started to produce penicillin, which was used widely during the World War II in soldiers with pneumonia and infected wounds. In the mid-1940s, penicillin became available for patients, and newspapers of the era nicknamed it "the miracle drug." Much later, scientists discovered how penicillin actually works: it stops bacteria from making their cell wall.

cosal membranes and cause fungal infections, such as vaginitis, or other, pathogenic bacteria may take over, such as *C. difficile*, which causes diarrhea and a potentially dangerous condition in the colon called pseudomembranous colitis.

The first antibiotic, penicillin, was discovered and made available around the time of World War II (see box), and then a race began among pharmaceutical companies to discover and produce more antibiotics. The industry poured a great deal of resources into this effort and, as a result, dozens of antibiotics are available today.

Antibiotics completely changed the face of modern medicine: they have cured millions of ill people all over the world and have contributed impressively to lengthening human life expectancy. In the preantibiotic era, nine of every ten children with bacterial meningitis died, and the one survivor likely lived with severe consequences, such as deafness or mental retardation. Strep throat (medically called streptococcal pharyngitis and tonsillitis) often damaged the heart, causing rheumatic fever, or led to death. Ear infections sometimes developed severe complications like meningitis or infection in the brain. Tuberculosis was rampant, attacking the lungs and other parts of the body and killing many of its victims. Pneumonias and whooping cough were dreaded and dangerous diseases, too. Today, every one of these illnesses can be effectively treated with antibiotics.

In discussing what antibiotics are, I have to stress what antibiotics are *not*. They are not active against viruses. Viruses are very small microorganisms, millionths of a millimeter in size. They are much smaller than bacteria, which are thousandths of a millimeter. Viruses cause a multitude of illnesses such as common cold, influenza, and most sore throats and coughs in children. Viruses also cause measles, chickenpox, mumps, hepatitis, AIDS, and many other diseases. The structure of viruses is completely different from the structure of bacteria. Thus, no matter how potent an antibacterial antibiotic is, it cannot kill a virus and cannot treat a viral infection. If you give your child an antibiotic when she has, for example, a viral respiratory infection, the antibiotic will not only have no effect on your child's symptoms, it may cause side effects for your child and contribute to making bacteria resistant to antibiotics.

What Is Microbial Resistance to Antibiotics?

Soon after the initial use of penicillin, doctors noticed that in some cases, the antibiotic was no longer active against bacteria such as *Staphylococcus*, which mainly causes skin infections like impetigo, boils, cellulitis, and abscesses. *Staphylococcus* had developed resistance to penicillin.

Since then, more and more bacteria have developed resistance to newer and stronger antibiotics. Infections caused by these resistant bacteria have become increasingly difficult to treat. In fact, the problem of microbial resistance to antibiotics is a critical problem in medicine and public health today.

How do germs develop resistance to antibiotics? As germs—and all organisms, including humans—reproduce, there are mutations, or random errors, that occur in their genetic material. Some of these mutations may allow the germ to survive in the presence of an antibiotic. For example, a mutation may change a germ's structure so that the antibiotic can no longer get through its cell wall to kill it. Thus, the resistant germ survives and passes its new ability to its offspring.

Because germs reproduce quickly, in a matter of hours or days, the number of resistant germs increases rapidly. Mutations are chance events, so resistance to an antibiotic can develop even without exposure to the drug. However, if the drug is present, it acts as a selection factor—think of a sieve—to block (kill) all the sensitive germs and allow only the resistant germs to reproduce. This scenario is an example of natural selection at work: the fittest germs are selected to survive and reproduce more and more of the resistant germs. It is a case of survival of the fittest.

There are three basic mechanisms that allow germs to become resistant to drugs:

1. They become impermeable to the drug or find a mechanism to push the drug out.
2. They change their protein receptors, to which the drug can no longer bind.
3. They produce enzymes that break down the drug.

Not all germs can develop resistance. For various reasons, some germs are not as "smart" as others. For example, group A *Streptococcus*, the bacterium that causes strep throat, has remained sensitive to penicillin, despite being exposed to this antibiotic for decades. The bacterium that causes syphilis, *Treponema pallidum*, has also remained sensitive to penicillin. However, these germs are the exceptions. Most germs have developed ways to become resistant and find new ways to survive exposure to new antibiotics.

Germs are ever resourceful. For example, they can share with each other, even from one species to another, the genetic material that gives them resistance. Resistant germs can remain in a person's body for weeks or even months, and even if they do not make the person ill, they can spread to other people, such as family members or classmates. For example, think of a child in a day care who takes antibiotics for an infection and ends up with antibiotic-resistant germs in her nose and throat. She puts a toy into her mouth and then another child touches the toy before putting his hand in his mouth. He now carries the resistant germ, too.

Imagine that those germs are *Pneumococcus* bacteria, which cause pneumonia, meningitis, and ear infections, and imagine that the little boy gets an ear infection from them. *Pneumococcus* used to be very sensitive to penicillin, but it no longer is because of the widespread use of penicillin over many years. *Pneumococcus* is also often resistant to many cephalosporins, which are antibiotics that work in a similar way to penicillin. The effective antibiotic options against this germ have decreased dramatically. The result is that the little boy's ear infection is difficult to treat. Now imagine how much more difficult it would be to treat a more serious illness, like pneumonia or meningitis.

It is not necessary to use only our imaginations. The problem of antibiotic resistance received extensive media attention in the summer of 2007 when a patient with multi-drug-resistant tuberculosis traveled from the United States to the Greek islands and back again, potentially exposing other passengers on air flights to the antibiotic-resistant mycobacteria that caused his illness.

Despite the larger number of antibiotics available today, doctors now have fewer therapeutic options in their arsenal to treat serious bacterial infections. Infections can last longer and give rise to complications as doctors try to treat them with one ineffective antibiotic after another. Most infections contracted while in the hospital are caused by multi-drug-resistant germs, making it more and more difficult to treat them and resulting in complications, prolonged hospital stays, and even deaths. Patients with weakened immune defenses are at particular risk from these resistant germs. Even healthy children and adults are susceptible to dangerous infections from common germs that have become difficult to treat, like MRSA (methicillin-resistant *Staphylococcus aureus*).

Scientists and doctors used to believe that humans would win over germs, because the pharmaceutical industry could continue to produce new antibiotics. However, this view does not seem to hold any longer. It has become slower and more difficult to develop antibiotics that can circumvent the increasingly more complex ways in which germs evade drugs. Germs are taking over the race.

What Constitutes Antibiotic Overuse?

In the past, doctors commonly prescribed an antibiotic when a patient had symptoms of a viral infection such as the common cold. Many physicians used the rationale that even if the antibiotic had no action against the virus, it would act against bacteria that might multiply while the patient's immune system was battling the virus. What could be the downside of such a practice? Both the parents and the doctor felt reassured that they had something to offer the sick child. Today, however, we know that this rationale is faulty; the excessive use of antibiotics has had a steep price, namely, the development of resistance among germs.

Some studies have found startling evidence of excessive antibiotic use. For example, in the 1990s, about 50 of 150 million antibiotic prescriptions, or one-third of all prescriptions, given to U.S. patients each year were for viral, not bacterial, infections. Another study in the United States found that, as recently as a few years ago, one-half of patients who went to their doctor with a common cold received a prescription for antibiotics.

This problem occurs in other parts of the world, too. In southern European countries antibiotic overuse is widespread, particularly the overuse of new, wide-spectrum, potent antibiotics. By contrast, in many northern European countries the most commonly used antibiotics are older, narrow-spectrum ones. This decision to use narrow-spectrum antibiotics rather than wide-spectrum ones is a factor that has contributed to the lower frequency of resistance to newer antibiotics in some Scandinavian countries.

In addition to the antibiotics that an individual is exposed to when taking them for an infection, everyone is exposed to antibiotics in the environment. Only a fraction of an antibiotic is actually metabolized by a patient's body, while the remainder is excreted in urine, which goes into the sewage system. Most sewage treatment facilities do not remove pharmaceutical products from the sewage stream, so antibiotics and other drugs are released with the treated sewage into the water supply. In addition, people often pour expired antibiotics down the drain, contributing to the pharmaceuticals in sewage, or discard them into waste containers where they end up in landfills. Water and soil tests frequently detect antibiotics, sometimes at levels high enough to treat infections.

People are also exposed to antibiotics through animals destined for human consumption, such as cattle, swine, poultry, and fish. Many farmers add antibiotics to animal feed to enhance the animals' growth, health, and weight. Studies estimate that over 70 percent of the antibiotics given to animals in the United States are to enhance growth rather than to treat infections. Some of the antibiotics are excreted into the soil, making their way to manure, environmental runoff, and the water supply, and some of the antibiotics go into animal flesh that people then eat.

Many European countries have forbidden the use of antibiotics as a growth factor in animal feed, but in the United States this practice continues, with obvious financial benefits for several parties involved. Organic meat products come from animals that have not been fed with antibiotics. Studies in both the United States and Europe have shown beyond doubt that using antibiotics in animal feed is closely correlated with antibiotic resistance in germs that affect humans.

Fortunately, there is some good news. Many doctors have become aware of the antibiotic-resistance problem and are now more careful in their prescribing habits. A few years ago, CDC started a large-scale campaign to re-educate doctors about the proper use of antibiotics, both within and outside hospitals. Already this effort seems to have been worthwhile. Recent data show that U.S. doctors have written about 40 percent fewer antibiotic prescriptions for children with common upper respiratory tract infections compared with the 1990s.

Similar efforts in Finland and other European countries have shown encouraging results: the frequency of germs resistant to a particular antibiotic seems to go down after using the antibiotic less. In addition, by avoiding antibiotics to treat viral infections, the percentage of resistant germs in the nose and throat of children declined tenfold.

The problem of antibiotic overuse is far from being resolved, however.

Everybody needs to take an active role. Therefore, infectious diseases specialists need to educate doctors in all specialties about the appropriate use of antibiotics. Doctors need to change their habits so that they prescribe antibiotics only when they are necessary, as well as educate parents—and patients in general—about appropriate antibiotic use. Parents need to understand that antibiotics will do nothing for their child's viral infections, the majority of common childhood ailments. The pharmaceutical industry (possibly with the help of government incentives) needs to limit its practice of promoting the wide use of newer and stronger antibiotics, which contributes to widespread resistance to these new antibiotics. (In fact, most nonserious bacterial infections can be treated with the older, narrow-spectrum antibiotics.) Finally, the government needs to establish national guidelines for antibiotic use in hospitals and doctors' offices, as well as incentives for the food production industry to use antibiotics more prudently.

What Are the Side Effects of Antibiotics?

Like any medication, antibiotics can have side effects. The most common side effects for children (and for adults) are gastrointestinal problems and allergic reactions. Gastrointestinal problems include stomachache, nausea, and diarrhea. About one in every five individuals treated with an antibiotic experiences diarrhea, which results from the antibiotic disrupting the microbial balance in the intestine. In other words, the antibiotic has killed not only the bacterium causing the infection but also microorganisms that help with food digestion and absorption. Narrow-spectrum antibiotics cause less widespread destruction of harmless and often necessary microbes. In some cases, antibiotic-related diarrhea can evolve into a severe colitis caused by the bacterium *C. difficile*, which produces toxins. Eating yogurt that contains beneficial microbes called probiotics can decrease the likelihood of antibiotic-related diarrhea.

Allergic reactions to antibiotics occur most commonly with penicillin and sulfonamides (sulfa drugs), but also with other antibiotics. Most allergic reactions to antibiotics are mild, typically with a skin rash, often accompanied by itching. Less often, a person experiences hives, difficulty in breathing, wheezing, or swelling in the face or throat that can cause difficulty swallowing. If your child develops any of these symptoms, take her to the doctor's office or the emergency room right away. Allergic reactions usually occur days or weeks after the first time a person takes a particular antibiotic. However, if the person takes the same antibiotic again, the allergic reaction can occur within minutes or a few hours. Rarely, an anaphylactic reaction occurs, causing a drop in blood pressure and shock. Anaphylactic reactions to penicillin happen about one time in every five thousand exposures to the drug.

Even though 15 percent or more of the population claims to be allergic to one or more antibiotics, only about 5 percent truly are allergic. Many people erroneously believe that nausea, vomiting, diarrhea, or other symptoms from taking an antibiotic indicate an allergy. They do not. Nevertheless, even with 5 percent of the population allergic to an antibiotic, the estimated 11 million times per year that U.S. children are prescribed antibiotics for a common cold translates into over five hundred thousand allergic reactions from unnecessary use of antibiotics.

Some antibiotics have additional side effects, as well as potentially dangerous interactions with other medications. For example, tetracycline antibiotics given to children younger than 8 years can cause tooth discoloration. Quinolones, one of the newer antibiotic classes, may cause damage to the bones, joints, and cartilage in young children, although this effect is still debated.

Recently, some studies have suggested that young children who are repeatedly exposed to antibiotics have an increased risk of developing asthma or other allergic disorders, as well as conditions like breast cancer in later life. Some data support this contention, but to date, these data are insufficient to confirm it. In terms of asthma risk, it is unclear whether a cause and effect link exists. Yes, some children who develop asthma received many antibiotics at a young age. But did the antibiotics cause the asthma? Perhaps the first symptoms of asthma were already beginning in the child and a doctor mistook them as upper respiratory infections and erroneously prescribed antibiotics. Or perhaps the child had viral respiratory infections that themselves later caused the asthma. Clearly, the relationship between antibiotics administered at a young age and later development of asthma has yet to be deciphered.

In terms of antibiotics and breast cancer, a U.S. study published in

2004 showed that women with breast cancer had had greater exposure to antibiotics over the many years prior to their diagnosis than women without breast cancer. However, this relationship was not statistically strong and does not prove that the increased exposure to antibiotics caused the breast cancer. Many more studies are needed to determine whether there really is a link.

Finally, some adolescents take antibiotics for prolonged periods because of severe acne, yet studies have shown no negative consequences for their later health. Given the scientific information to date, I strongly recommend that you not become overly concerned about your children taking antibiotics if they need them. Even if they need to take three, four, or five courses of antibiotics in their first few years of life, which can happen for children susceptible to ear or throat infections, it's better that they take the antibiotics to resolve the infections. Of course, as I discussed earlier, your children should take only antibiotics prescribed by a doctor for bacterial infections. More on when and how to give antibiotics to your children in a moment.

Can Antibiotics Prevent an Infection?

Antibiotics are used mainly to treat infections that have already begun, but sometimes doctors prescribe them to prevent infections from beginning in the first place. These cases are specific and limited, and because of the antibiotic resistance problem, using antibiotics for preventive reasons has markedly decreased. However, using antibiotics preventively is valid in certain instances.

Some children get frequent urinary tract infections, and their doctor may administer antibiotics to decrease the frequency of such infections. Antibiotics are also given to patients with rheumatic fever to prevent recurrences. Family members might be given antibiotics because of their close contact with a person sick with particular dangerous germs, such as *Meningococcus* or pertussis (whooping cough). Children with some immune defects, sickle cell disease, or those who have had their spleen removed need to take preventive antibiotics, as do children bitten by a dog or other animal. In addition, some patients may need to take preventive antibiotics before certain surgical or dental procedures.

In each of these cases, there is a higher than normal chance of a person contracting an infection. Otherwise healthy children who happen to have a cold should not be given antibiotics to prevent an ear infection or pneumonia.

Are There Antimicrobials against Other Germs?

The scientific progress in developing antibiotics against bacteria has not been matched for treating viral, fungal, or parasitic infections. The development of antimicrobials against these kinds of germs has been slower. There are antivirals against only a few viruses: influenza, some herpes viruses, hepatitis B and C viruses, and HIV. Incidentally, antiviral drug research received a great boost by the HIV epidemic, which promoted intense research activity and advanced the development of antiviral drugs for more viruses than just HIV.

For other viruses, including those that cause polio, measles, mumps, rubella, and chickenpox, there are vaccines but no antivirals. Vaccines prevent most cases of these diseases, but they do not treat them in infected people. I discuss vaccines further in chapter 9.

For some viruses, there is neither vaccine nor antiviral treatment. This is the case with most viruses that cause common childhood infections, such as common colds and diarrheas. Another example is the more serious respiratory syncytial virus, or RSV, which causes bronchiolitis, an inflammation of the small airways, and which sickens or kills many young children in the United States and all over the world.

Even available antiviral drugs do not eradicate the viral infection in the same way that antibacterial drugs do for bacterial infections. Rather, most antivirals decrease the length of time that a person experiences symptoms, lessen the seriousness of symptoms, and reduce the frequency of complications. Antivirals also make the illness in the treated person less contagious. They are only used in certain circumstances. Antivirals against influenza are most useful if given within one or two days of flu symptoms beginning. Flu antivirals are reserved for people with increased risk of severe illness, such as very young children, the elderly, people with immune suppression, and people with some preexisting diseases.

Fungi include yeasts and molds, many of which are harmless to humans. Some fungi can cause infections, however, when their spores are inhaled or enter the body through a skin injury. Several antifungal creams, ointments, and shampoos are available to treat superficial fungal infections of the skin or nails, which affect healthy adults and children. Sometimes, immunosuppressed patients or premature infants contract a serious, whole-body fungal infection, for which there are some antifungal drugs. The pharmaceutical industry is becoming more interested in developing antifungals given the growing number and longer survival of patients with weakened immune systems, including people with HIV/AIDS, people undergoing chemotherapy, and transplant recipients.

Last, parasites are microorganisms that range in size from slightly larger than bacteria, such as the malaria-causing *Plasmodium*, to visible with the naked eye, such as worms. Parasites are a major problem worldwide, causing billions of cases of illness and deaths, particularly in the developing world. Yet few antiparasitic drugs are available. Progress in this area has not advanced at an equal pace to progress with antibacterial and antiviral drugs.

Antimicrobial drugs against viruses, fungi, and parasites are not immune to the drug resistance problem that is so prevalent with bacteria. These other kinds of germs can and do develop resistance to antimicrobials. For example, some of the drugs against influenza and other viruses have become obsolete because of resistant viruses.

How Are Antibiotics Used Appropriately?

If your child's doctor prescribes an antibiotic, make sure that she takes it correctly:

- Follow the doctor's instructions for the recommended number of doses per day and the recommended duration of treatment.
- Complete the full course of antibiotics, even if your child feels better after taking the antibiotic for only a few days. Scientists believe that stopping an antibiotic too early allows some germs to survive, even though in smaller numbers, and to begin growing again. The result could be another infection, complications from

the initial infection, or mutations in the germ that lead to antibiotic resistance.

- Don't give your child an antibiotic that has been prescribed for another person, even if her symptoms are similar, or an antibiotic left over from a previous prescription. These antibiotics may not be the right ones, may have expired, or may be inadequate for a full course.
- Tell the doctor if your child does not show signs of improvement after three or four days of antibiotic treatment. It could be that the germ causing the infection is resistant to the particular antibiotic, and your child may have to try a different one.
- Give your child yogurt to eat while she is on the antibiotic. Many yogurts contain cultures of good microbes, called probiotics, which can decrease the chances of antibiotic-related diarrhea.

As I have noted, antibiotics work against bacterial infections, not viral infections. If your child is ill and you are concerned about her, take her to your pediatrician to determine whether her infection is caused by a bacterium or a virus. Distinguishing between the two can be tricky, but in most cases a doctor will be able to do so. See also the box in this chapter describing symptoms of a viral cold and a bacterial sinus infection.

In general, viruses in children cause colds; most cases of bronchitis (coughing), sore throat, and runny nose; many cases of pneumonia; and some cases of ear infection. None of these viral infections can be treated

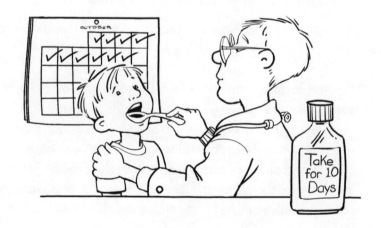

How Does a Cold Differ from a Sinus Infection?

It is sometimes difficult to tell the difference between a cold, which is a viral infection that gets better on its own, and a sinus infection (sinusitis), which is a bacterial infection treated with antibiotics for at least ten days. The American Academy of Pediatrics provides the following guidance for parents.

In general, the signs and symptoms of a viral cold include the following:

At the beginning, nasal discharge is clear.

After two days, nasal discharge becomes thicker and white, yellow, or green.

After a few more days, nasal discharge becomes clear again and dries up.

Usually a cough occurs, and it may get worse at night.

Sometimes, a fever occurs, usually at the beginning of the cold. Most of the time, the fever is low and lasts for only one to two days.

Symptoms peak after three to five days and then improve and slowly disappear over the next seven to ten days.

The signs and symptoms of a bacterial sinus infection may include the following:

Cold symptoms last for more than ten days without *improvement.*

A fever lasts for at least three or four days in a row.

Nasal discharge is thick and yellow.

A severe headache occurs around the eyes and gets worse when bending over.

Swelling and dark circles may appear around the eyes and are worse in the morning.

Bad breath occurs along with cold symptoms. (However, bad breath can also be a sign of a sore throat or simply that a child is not brushing her teeth.)

If your child develops a severe headache, pain in the back of the neck, swelling and redness around the eyes, persistent vomiting, irritability, and sensitivity to light, you should immediately seek medical help. In very rare cases, a bacterial sinus infection may spread to the eye or the brain and its coverings.

with antibiotics. Yet in the United States, up to three-quarters of antibiotic prescriptions for children are given to "treat" these very infections. Why? One factor is parental pressure. Parents often believe that antibiotics will help their child. One of the best things you can do as a parent is to listen to the doctor's recommended treatment, and if it doesn't include antibiotics, don't demand them. In addition, do not make the decision yourself to give your children antibiotics.

--- | MAIN POINTS | ---
Measures to Use Antibiotics Appropriately

- Keep in mind that antibiotics are active against bacteria and have no effect against viruses.
- Know that viruses cause the majority of routine infections in children (colds, runny nose, cough, sore throat, diarrhea).
- Be aware of antibiotics' side effects, including gastrointestinal upset and allergic reactions.
- Don't contribute to antibiotic overuse, which leads to germs developing resistance to antibiotics. When germs are resistant, the antibiotics lose their effect.
- Use antibiotics judiciously, because this worthwhile effort can make germs sensitive to antibiotics again.
- Don't give your child antibiotics without your doctor's recommendation. Always follow instructions about dosing and duration of an antibiotic course.

9

The Miracle of Modern Prevention

VACCINE SAFETY AND EFFECTIVENESS

Few discoveries have changed human history and life expectancy so dramatically as the discovery of vaccines. As recently as two generations ago, when my grandparents were young children, childhood was very different than it is today. In the decades before the 1950s, most children became sick with infections like measles, rubella, and chickenpox. These infections were extremely common, and some children developed severe complications from them or even died. More dangerous infections, such as whooping cough and diphtheria, claimed the lives of many children. Poliomyelitis crippled or killed thousands of children every year. Even chickenpox—an illness that I and most of my generation had as children—caused serious problems for the skin, lungs, or brain of one in thirty children, and one in three hundred died (yes, from chickenpox). When the children's hospital of my alma mater, Johns Hopkins University, opened in 1912, it had separate buildings to isolate children with infections. They were full of children with poliomyelitis, diphtheria, measles, and mumps. Of course, this situation continues today in hospitals in many African countries and in other parts of the developing world.

If you could have told someone one hundred years ago that these devastating childhood infections would be almost eliminated in the near future, he would have probably dismissed the notion as science fiction. Yet this very situation has been achieved today. Thanks to the discovery of vaccines and their wide implementation, one dreadful disease, smallpox, has been eradicated from the world; another one, poliomyelitis, has been eliminated from the Western Hemisphere; and other diseases have become so rare that even doctors have seen only a handful of cases. During my training in the 1990s in pediatrics and pediatric infectious diseases at three hospitals in the United States, I saw only one or two cases of measles. Today, most children and parents in resource-rich countries live without the fear and worries of these childhood illnesses, thanks to vaccinations.

In this chapter, I describe what vaccines are, how they work, and which vaccines children in the United States should get. I include some information for parents of children with a preexisting medical condition, such as a weakened immune system. I also discuss the possible side effects from vaccines, including the controversy and claims that have spread about supposed serious effects of certain vaccines.

What Are Vaccines and Why Should Children Be Vaccinated?

A vaccine is a biological preparation that gives a person immunity to a particular disease, meaning that the immune system acquires the ability to resist the disease. Thus, vaccines prevent infectious diseases and their consequences. Vaccines are made with microorganisms, like bacteria or viruses, that are either dead (inactivated) or live and attenuated (weakened). Some vaccines are made with parts of microorganisms, like their proteins or inactivated toxins.

Like any other medication or medical intervention, vaccines are not 100 percent effective. However, most vaccines are between 85 percent and 95 percent effective, and they protect the great majority of vaccinated children from the potentially serious consequences of many infectious diseases. Some vaccines are administered alone, while others are combined, such as the measles-mumps-rubella (MMR) vaccine combination. Some vaccines provide lifelong immunity, while others require periodic booster doses to "top up" a person's immunity. More in a moment on how vaccines actually work.

In the developed world, the wide use of vaccines in children has reduced by over 90 percent the cases of vaccine-preventable infectious diseases, diseases that caused epidemics in the past. Some people are highly critical about the safety of vaccines, but they do not talk about the huge benefits that vaccination has brought to child survival and quality of life. Indeed, it is ironic that because of vaccines, we have forgotten the severe complications and devastating consequences of many childhood diseases. Most parents today have never heard the sound of whooping cough, and they have not seen how serious an illness it can be for a young baby. They have not seen a child paralyzed by polio or a child die from measles.

Many people believe that because these and other vaccine-preventable diseases are now rare in the West, it is no longer necessary to have their children vaccinated. In other words, they think their children are not at risk of contracting one of these diseases. This thinking is incorrect. The reason that vaccine-preventable diseases are rare is because the vast majority of people are immunized against these diseases. If the level of immunization in a community declines by even a small amount, infections that had become extremely rare soon return.

With the exception of smallpox and, in the West only, polio, the germs that cause all infectious diseases continue to live and circulate at very low levels. People who are not immune do contract these diseases, so the greater the number of people who are not immune, the greater the outbreak and spread becomes. In addition, the germs of infectious diseases exist in high concentrations in countries where immunization levels are low, and these countries are only an airplane ride away.

The kind of incorrect thinking I just described, along with false and exaggerated claims about vaccine side effects (which I discuss later), may have led to a small decline in immunization against measles, mumps, and rubella in the United States in recent years. As a result, in 2008, more cases of measles were reported than during the entire previous decade. About 3 to 4 million cases of measles and approximately 450 deaths from measles used to occur every year in the United States before immunization was introduced in 1963. With widespread immunization, the number of cases has decreased to fewer than 100 per year, with most of them having a link to an imported case and occurring among unvaccinated children. Since 2005, measles cases have also risen in Europe, again a result of decreasing levels of immunization in children. In addition to

How Was Vaccination Discovered?

About two hundred years ago, farmers in England observed that milkmaids did not contract smallpox if they had already been infected with a much milder pox virus, called *Vaccinia*, that makes cows sick. In 1796, an English physician, Edward Jenner, decided to test this observation with an experiment. He took pus from the skin blister of a milkmaid who had the *Vaccinia* virus and inserted it in a young child's skin. A few weeks later, he repeated this procedure on the child, but this time he added a small amount of material from a smallpox blister. The child did not contract smallpox. Jenner repeated the experiment in other individuals, and none of them became sick with smallpox either.

Jenner created the term *vaccination* from the Latin word *vacca*, meaning cow, and presented his results to the Royal Academy of London. Thus, medicine changed dramatically as a result of a piece of local knowledge given by English farmers to a physician who was willing to listen and carefully examine the knowledge.

The next leap of progress in vaccination occurred decades later, when Louis Pasteur in France proved that a disease can be prevented in an individual who has been previously infected with weakened germs. In 1855, he used a vaccine that he had prepared with weakened rabies virus to prevent rabies in a boy who had been bitten by a rabid dog. The vaccine was successful and paved the way for the microbial theory, which states that every infection is caused by a specific germ. Many people had suspected this theory to be true, but it was not generally accepted at the time.

The great progress in vaccination that we benefit from today occurred in the mid-twentieth century with the discovery of vaccines against polio, tetanus, diphtheria, pertussis, measles, and many others. The list of infections for which there is a vaccine continues to grow.

increasing the risk of contracting measles, not having the MMR vaccine leaves young women vulnerable to rubella during pregnancy, with potentially devastating consequences for the fetus.

There are more examples of vaccine-preventable diseases rearing their heads again in developed countries. The number of cases of pertussis, or whooping cough, has been increasing both in the United States and in Europe, because too few adolescents and adults get their booster dose of the pertussis vaccine. Therefore, they lose their immunity and become susceptible to the disease. If they then become sick with whooping cough, they risk spreading it to young infants, who are very susceptible to its harmful consequences, including pneumonia and encephalitis (brain inflammation).

The risks from vaccine-preventable infectious diseases are real and will quickly magnify if childhood immunization declines or stops. Many of the vaccine-preventable illnesses are more severe in adults than in children, chickenpox being one example. By not immunizing our children when they are young, we leave them vulnerable to more serious illness in their adult years. Not vaccinating carries risks both for your child and, if your child becomes ill, for other people who may be exposed to your child, including people with cancer and others with a weak immune system.

Which Vaccines Are Recommended for U.S. Children?

Each country has its own schedule of childhood immunizations, depending on economic factors, microbial risks specific to its geography and socioeconomic level, and the willingness of public health authorities to establish the necessary programs. In the United States, vaccines that target fifteen microorganisms are recommended for all children. In many states, children cannot start day care or kindergarten if they have not received the recommended vaccinations. Exceptions are allowed in the case of religious or other objections to vaccines, but if there is an outbreak of a vaccine-preventable disease, an unimmunized child must stay home from day care or school for days or weeks.

The recommended vaccines are

- hepatitis B
- rotavirus
- diphtheria, tetanus, and pertussis (given as a combined vaccine), abbreviated to DTaP (The "a" stands for acellular pertussis vaccine.)

- *Hemophilus influenzae* type B
- *Pneumococcus*
- poliomyelitis
- influenza
- measles, mumps, and rubella (given as a combined vaccine), abbreviated to MMR
- varicella (chickenpox)
- hepatitis A
- *Meningococcus*

In general, children receive these immunizations in their first two years of life according to a schedule produced by the American Academy of Pediatrics (table 9.1). This schedule (and the vaccine dose) has been determined after careful consideration of many factors, including a vaccine's safety and effectiveness, and is designed to provide the maximum possible preventive benefit.

If your children do not receive the recommended vaccines at the recommended ages, they remain at risk from the particular disease and can place others at risk also. Do not delay your children's vaccinations, and do not give less than the recommended doses. Many of the vaccine-preventable diseases can strike at an early age and are often more serious when they affect an infant or young child than when they affect older children, an example being whooping cough (pertussis). If your children have fallen behind with some immunizations, in most cases they can continue where they left off and will not have to start from the beginning.

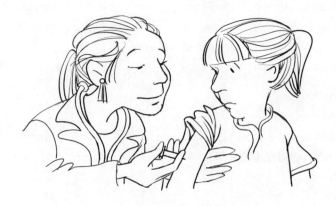

TABLE 9.1

Recommended immunization schedule from birth to 6 years in the United States

Vaccine	Birth	1 month	2 months	4 months	6 months	12 months	15 months	18 months	19 to 23 months	2 to 3 years	4 to 6 years
Hepatitis B	HepB	HepB			HepB						
Rotavirus			RV	RV	RV						
Diphtheria, tetanus, pertussis			DTaP	DTaP	DTaP		DTaP				DTaP
Haemophilus influenzae type b			Hib	Hib	Hib	Hib					
Pneumococcal			PCV	PCV	PCV	PCV				PPSV	
Inactivated poliovirus			IPV	IPV	IPV	IPV					IPV
Influenza					Influenza (yearly)						
Measles, mumps, rubella						MMR					MMR
Varicella						Varicella					Varicella
Hepatitis A						HepA (2 doses)				HepA series	
Meningococcal										MCV (2 doses) series	

DTaP: diphtheria-tetanus-acellular pertussis; PCV: pneumococcal conjugate vaccine; PPSV: pneumococcal polysaccharide vaccine; IPV: inactivated poliomyelitis vaccine; MCV: meningoccal conjugate vaccine; MMR: measles, mumps, rubella.

▢ Range of recommended ages for all children except certain high-risk groups

▢ Range of recommended ages for certain high-risk groups

TABLE 9.2
The recommended immunization schedule from ages 7 to 18 in the United States

Vaccine	Age		
	7 to 10 years	11 to 12 years	13 to 18 years
Tetanus, diphtheria, pertussis		Tdap	Tdap
Human papillomavirus		HPV (3 doses)	HPV series
Meningococcal	MCV (2 doses)	MCV series	MCV series
Influenza		Influenza (yearly)	
Pneumococcal		PPSV	
Hepatitis A		HepA series	
Hepatitis B		HepB series	
Inactivated poliovirus		IPV series	
Measles, mumps, rubella		MMR series	
Varicella		Varicella series	

MCV: meningococcal conjugate vaccine; Tdap: tetanus-diphtheria (adult)-acellular pertussis; PPSV: pneumococcal polysaccharide vaccine; IPV: inactivated poliomyelitis vaccine.
▓ Range of recommended ages for all children except certain high-risk groups
▓ Range of recommended ages for catch-up immunization
▓ Range of recommended ages for certain high-risk groups

During the toddler and school years and into adolescence, children receive booster doses of some previously administered vaccines, as shown in table 9.2. A recent addition is a vaccine against human papilloma virus (HPV), which protects against cervical cancer and is recommended for girls 11 years of age or older. The need for adolescents to receive vaccines is sometimes forgotten. Adolescents need the following:

- a booster dose of the Tdap vaccine
- the meningococcal vaccine
- the hepatitis B vaccine, if not previously vaccinated
- a second dose of the MMR vaccine if they didn't receive two doses during childhood
- the chickenpox vaccine if they haven't been immunized or haven't had the chickenpox illness
- the influenza vaccine every fall, particularly if they have a condition that places them at high risk for severe influenza, such as asthma or a heart condition, or if they have young siblings

Note that the influenza vaccine should be repeated every fall for *all* children over 6 months of age, as well as for parents of children younger than 2 years. The influenza virus changes continually, so one year's vaccine is not effective against the following year's influenza strains.

Other vaccines are recommended in particular cases. For example, yellow fever and typhoid fever vaccines are recommended before traveling to certain countries (see chapter 6 for more details). In some cases, the measles vaccine, which is normally given after the age of 12 months, can be given earlier, between 6 and 12 months, if a baby must travel to countries with a high risk for measles. In addition, a vaccine is sometimes required when a person is exposed to a particular disease, such as rabies from an animal bite.

A child with a mild illness such as a runny nose, a cough, an ear infection, or mild diarrhea can be vaccinated safely. A child taking antibiotics can also receive immunizations as normal. Children allergic to penicillin, amoxicillin, cephalosporins, or sulfonamides can receive all recommended vaccines. In addition, a baby being breastfed can receive all recommended vaccines, and the mother can be vaccinated while nursing, too. However, pregnant women should avoid vaccines that contain live microorganisms (MMR and chickenpox vaccines and the nasally administered flu vaccine). For more on pregnancy and vaccinations, see chapter 10.

I recommend that you keep a written record of all vaccines your children receive, as well as the dates they were given. If you move or change doctors, this information will make it easier to continue vaccinations so that your children remain fully protected from vaccine-preventable diseases. If you suspect that your child has any side effects after an immunization, let your doctor know, especially before another dose of the same vaccine is given to your child. Your doctor may report possible side effects to the national system of surveillance, which tracks possible vaccine side effects to ensure vaccine safety. I discuss vaccine safety in more detail later in this chapter.

The American Academy of Pediatrics and the Centers for Disease Control and Prevention (CDC) offer vaccine information for both parents and doctors (see www.aap.org/immunization and www.cdc.gov/vaccines). In addition, the Johns Hopkins University's renowned Institute for the

Safety of Vaccines (www.vaccinesafety.edu) independently assesses vaccines and their safety.

When Some Vaccines Should Be Avoided

The parents of a child with some medical conditions such as a history of prematurity or a weakened immune system may wonder if it is safe for their child to receive all the recommended vaccines. If your child was born prematurely, most of the vaccines, with only a few exceptions, can be given normally (according to the child's chronological age). In the case of a very small premature baby, your doctor will recommend what should be adjusted in the vaccination schedule.

Some children may have a condition or be on medication that weakens their immune system. For example, a child may have cancer, AIDS, or a congenital immunodeficiency; may be undergoing chemotherapy or taking corticosteroids; or may be an organ transplant recipient. In these cases, your doctor will advise you according to your child's specific circumstances and the balance of risk and benefit for each vaccination. In general, vaccines that contain live attenuated viruses or bacteria, such as the MMR and chickenpox vaccines and the nasal vaccine for influenza, should be avoided in children with a weakened immune system. Often, these vaccines can be administered once the immunosuppressing agent or therapy has been discontinued. If your children are in contact with an immunosuppressed individual in the household or at a day care, they can receive the vaccines for MMR and chickenpox as normal; the weakened virus in these vaccines does not spread disease to other individuals in contact with a vaccinated child.

Vaccines that contain inactivated or dead bacteria or viruses are safe to administer to immunosuppressed children, including the vaccines against diphtheria-tetanus-pertussis, hepatitis A, hepatitis B, polio, *haemophilus influenzae*, *Pneumococcus*, and *Meningococcus*, and the injectable flu vaccine. However, the vaccines may not be as effective, because the immune system of such individuals is suppressed and may not be able to produce sufficient immunity. In some instances, steroids do not affect the immune system substantially, so vaccines can be administered normally. These instances include when steroids are given at a low dose, are given by mouth for less than two weeks, or are given by a different route (not by mouth), such as on the skin, as a spray, or in an inhaler.

Particular vaccines should be avoided in a few other instances:

- If your child had a severe reaction to a previous dose of a vaccine, such as an anaphylactic reaction with hives, difficulty breathing, facial swelling, or a drop in blood pressure, the particular vaccine should not be administered again.
- If your child has a severe allergy to eggs, the injectable flu vaccine should not be administered.
- If your child has a neurological disorder with seizures or other symptoms and the cause of the disorder is not known, then the pertussis vaccine can be postponed until the disorder is further defined.
- If your child takes aspirin for chronic arthritis, takes chronic corticosteroids by mouth, or has asthma, the live flu vaccine (nasally administered) should be avoided. Instead, he should receive the inactivated flu vaccine (injectable).
- If your child is sick with a high fever, immunizations should be postponed until his illness resolves. This precaution is necessary because it is otherwise difficult to know whether the fever and other symptoms are due to the illness or to a possible reaction to the vaccine.

Finally, in the rare case that your child has an allergy to latex or to the additives or preservatives that may be contained in vaccines, you should discuss the situation with your doctor.

How Do Vaccines Work?

Vaccines work by giving a person immunity, which is to say by giving a person's immune system the ability to resist a particular disease. The immune system is responsible for the body's defense against invaders like germs. To clarify how vaccines work in the immune system, I will start this discussion with a brief introduction to the field of immunology.

When a person is infected by a germ, be it a bacterium or a virus, his immune system is activated and attracts white blood cells to the site of the infection. For example, in a skin infection, white blood cells would go to the affected area in the skin, or in a respiratory infection, to the respiratory mucosal membranes. Some white blood cells, called *phagocytes*, kill germs directly by engulfing, or swallowing, them or by producing chemical toxins to attack them. Other white blood cells, the *lymphocytes*, produce special proteins called antibodies to locate the invader, bind to it—like a key in a lock—and lead it away to be destroyed by the phagocytic cells.

It takes time for white blood cells to defeat germs, so the germs will have had a chance to cause symptoms in the infected person. In some cases, the immune system's counterattack is not very quick or dynamic, leading to a severe or even a lethal infection. In the majority of cases, however, the body's counterattack eradicates the invader, and the symptoms resolve.

Once the germs have been destroyed, the antibodies that were produced to combat the germs remain in the body in small quantities, ready to be activated if the same germ makes a repeat invasion. For this reason, someone who had measles or chickenpox during childhood is immune to the disease and will not get sick again, even if he is re-exposed. The lymphocytes that became activated the first time are ready to neutralize the invader, and they act much more rapidly on subsequent exposures, before the germ has a chance to multiply and cause symptoms. This phenomenon is called *immunologic memory* and lasts for many years, often for the rest of our lives. The body's defenses can decline, however, and make someone vulnerable to these invaders again in situations like a person living to a very advanced age; having certain diseases, such as cancer; or taking some medications in large doses, such as corticosteroids or cancer chemotherapy.

Vaccination is based on the principle of immunologic memory. Vaccines are made with one of three components: dead germs; live germs that have been attenuated, or weakened, in the laboratory; or germ products, like proteins or toxins. These components stimulate the immune system to produce antibodies for the particular germ in the vaccine. Thus, the body will be ready to face that germ if exposed to it. The immune system will have the necessary memory to quickly produce large amounts of the specific antibodies before the germ has time to multiply enough to cause disease.

Sometimes, more than one dose of a vaccine is necessary for the immune system to produce adequate antibodies or to produce antibodies that will last for a long time. For example, antibodies against the virus that causes measles last all our lives, but the antibodies against tetanus decline over time to very low levels. Therefore, people need to have a booster dose of the tetanus vaccine every seven to ten years. Some viruses, like influenza, mutate and change from year to year, so the antibodies produced by the immune system after one year's vaccination will not bind efficiently to the new virus strains circulating the following winter. For this reason, the influenza vaccine needs to be administered every year.

So far, I have been talking about active production of antibodies, meaning antibodies produced by a person's own immune system after vaccination. There is another way to acquire antibodies, however: through passive transfer. A newborn baby has partial protection against many infections thanks to antibodies that passed through the placenta from the mother's blood to the baby's blood circulation. This transfer of antibodies from mother to fetus happens during the last trimester of pregnancy. Because the baby received these antibodies through passive transfer rather than producing them himself, the level of antibodies declines rapidly during the first few months of life, making the baby vulnerable to his microbial environment.

To ensure that the baby remains protected against vaccine-preventable diseases, and because the risk of disease from many germs is highest during infancy, a baby's immunizations should begin during the first few months of life. For maximum effectiveness, it is critical that the vaccine schedule be followed and the vaccines be given at their recommended times.

Similar to the passive transfer of antibodies from mother to fetus, a person can receive passive immunization. Passive immunization consists of giving a person the actual antibodies (rather than the means of creating antibodies) against a particular germ. Certain situations require passive immunization. For example, if a child has not been immunized against the germ that causes a disease for which a vaccine exists and has not been exposed to the disease in the past, he has no antibodies against it. If he is now exposed to the disease, there is not enough time for him to receive the vaccine and produce his own antibodies. Therefore, he is given "premade" antibodies.

These premade antibodies come from human (or animal) blood that has immunity against the particular germ, or they are synthesized in a laboratory. Antibodies of human origin are usually called *antiserum* or *immune globulin*, or, when enriched in specific antibodies, *hyperimmune globulin*, and synthesized antibodies are usually *monoclonal antibodies* (named after the production technique). An example of an immune globulin from a human source is the tetanus immune globulin, which consists of antibodies against the tetanus toxin that can be given to a person with extensive or dirty wounds and inadequate immunization.

In another example, a person exposed to rabies from the bite of a rabid animal should receive the antirabies immune globulin, which is of human origin, along with the rabies vaccine. Monoclonal antibodies are used against respiratory syncytial virus (RSV) and are given preventively to premature babies and other babies with risk factors for serious RSV infection.

Passive immunization protects a person for only a short time—a few weeks to months—because the antibodies decay and are eliminated from the blood. In contrast, active immunization (vaccines) confers long-term and sometimes lifelong protection against the particular germs.

How Safe Are Vaccines?

You have undoubtedly read or heard about claims that vaccines can cause severe side effects. Conditions that have been attributed to vaccines, at one time or another, include damage to the developing brain, seizures, autism, and multiple sclerosis. Other claims are that vaccines contain dangerously high levels of mercury and that the large number of vaccines a child receives will weaken or confuse his immune system. Given this multitude of accusations, many parents understandably worry and are uncertain about whether they should immunize their children. Many independent scientific and medical entities have studied the claims extensively, however, and have reached conclusions based on the scientific and clinical data that are available. What, then, is the truth about vaccines?

Real Vaccine Risks

Before a vaccine can be made commercially available, it is tested extensively for safety and effectiveness. Scientists create vaccines in the laboratory and then test a vaccine in animal studies and subsequently in human studies. During this process, several thousand individuals are tested, and the vaccine must be proven effective and safe before its approval. Only once a vaccine has gone through rigorous testing and been approved can it be included in the schedule of recommended immunizations for children.

Many vaccines produce mild local side effects such as pain or light swelling and redness at the site of the injection. Infants may also develop a slight fever after several of the vaccines have been administered. For example, both the DTaP and the MMR vaccines can cause fever. In fact, a fever from the MMR vaccine usually develops a week after vaccination. A mild rash, sometimes accompanied by a slight fever, can also occur after some vaccines. For example, a rash may appear one week after the MMR vaccine or within one month after the chickenpox vaccine. Fever and other mild local symptoms usually resolve within a day or two without any negative consequences for a child's health. In a few cases, the reaction at the injection site can be more extensive, with pain or swelling, but it usually resolves without any further problems.

Unfortunately, there have been some cases of serious consequences after a vaccine, but such effects are very rare:

- After receiving an earlier version of the DTP vaccine (which did not have the acellular pertussis vaccine), fewer than one in one hundred children developed persistent high-pitched crying, excessive sleepiness, high fever, or seizures (usually as a result of the fever). These side effects are now less frequent, at less than one in ten thousand, with the new vaccine (DTaP), which does not contain whole cells of the pertussis bacterium.
- Encephalopathy, which is inflammation of the brain, happened extremely rarely (1 in 110,000 doses) after administering the early

pertussis vaccine. It is not known whether the vaccine caused this response or if another condition was responsible, such as an infection that happened to occur shortly after the vaccine was given. Long-term epidemiological studies have found no evidence of the pertussis vaccine causing brain damage. Today, the acellular pertussis vaccine is used in the United States; a very large, ten-year study of Canadian children has not found any relationship between the new acellular vaccine and permanent brain damage.

- About one of every six hundred thousand doses of hepatitis B vaccine causes a severe allergic reaction called *anaphylaxis*, with the person experiencing hives, difficulty breathing, or a drop in blood pressure. Nevertheless, no one has ever died from getting the hepatitis B vaccine, whereas thousands of people die every year soon after being infected with hepatitis B virus.

- The orally administered polio vaccine that used to be administered caused the rare side effect of paralysis in 1 in 750,000 doses. The injectable polio vaccine in use today completely avoids this side effect.

- Very rarely, the influenza and tetanus vaccines may cause a neurological disorder called Guillain-Barré syndrome, which can lead to paralysis. The incidence of this syndrome occurring after the flu vaccine is one in 1 million, so indeed very rare. Remember, also, that the risks from influenza and tetanus can occur more frequently than this rare potential side effect.

In the United States, as well as in other countries, there is a system in place for doctors to report illnesses that develop after giving a vaccine, even if the symptoms are not related to the vaccine. In this way, some rare potential adverse effects of a vaccine can be detected. For example, a few years ago, a vaccine against rotavirus, which causes intestinal infection and diarrhea, was approved in the United States for use in infants. The reporting system led to the discovery that for one in ten thousand infants vaccinated, this vaccine could cause a condition called *intussusception*. This condition, in which a fragment of the intestine inserts itself telescopically into another, is dangerous and often needs surgery. The complication occurred so rarely after vaccination with this particular rotavirus vaccine that it was impossible to detect during the initial clinical studies, which usually are performed on a few thousand individuals. It became evident only once the vaccine was approved for use and was administered to many thousands of people. The vaccine was withdrawn from use in the United States; a different vaccine against rotavirus is in use today. Most of the vaccines available today have been used for many years, so this accumulated experience provides a very accurate guide to their safety.

The Facts about Claims of Serious Vaccine Side Effects

When a particular condition develops after a person receives a vaccine, it can be difficult to determine whether the vaccine is to blame or whether the timing is coincidental. In some cases, a new condition may become apparent in a child very soon after a vaccine is administered, leading parents to believe that it might be related. Children receive vaccines several times during their first and second years of life. During these very same years, some conditions, like autism, may make their first appearance, or certain events, like sudden infant death syndrome, can occur. It is easy to understand why parents, devastated by a diagnosis or the sudden and incomprehensible death of their infant, may point fingers at a vaccine that their child received shortly before the event. Here is a look at the main claims that have been made about serious vaccine side effects.

There have been claims that the DTP vaccine can cause sudden infant death syndrome (SIDS). The first dose of this vaccine is given when a baby is 2 months old, which is also the time of highest risk for SIDS, a rare syndrome for which the causes are still unclear. Since the 1980s, many studies have examined a possible link between vaccination and SIDS. The studies consistently find that the number of SIDS cases among infants who have received the vaccine is the same as the number of SIDS cases that would be expected by chance alone. In addition, the number of infants receiving vaccines has increased, yet the frequency of sudden death in babies has decreased during the same time. The decline in SIDS cases began after the recommendation that babies sleep on their back.

Another claim states that the vaccine against MMR causes autism. Autism is a spectrum of developmental disorders that has increased in frequency over approximately the past twenty years. Often, autism is diagnosed during a child's second year of life, and some critics blamed the

MMR vaccine, which is administered between 12 to 15 months of age. A possible link was raised by a 1998 study from England that reported twelve cases of children diagnosed with developmental disorders or autism a few weeks after receiving the MMR vaccine. Needless to say, this study received extensive coverage by the mass media. However, the study was fraught with problems: it examined a very small number of patients, and it did not include comparison groups of children without autism who had received the vaccine or children who had not received the vaccine but developed autism. In addition, the proposed mechanism—that the intestinal mucosa is damaged and toxins from the measles virus pass through that way to the brain—has not been demonstrated scientifically.

Since this initial study, many others have reported results that do not support a relationship between the vaccine and autism. One of these studies, from Denmark, followed one hundred thousand children for over six years and found no difference in how frequently autism developed in children who received the vaccine compared with children who did not receive the vaccine. Also, the U.S. National Academy of Sciences asked the Institute of Medicine—an independent body of medical experts without ties of any kind to the companies that produce vaccines nor to the authorities that recommend vaccines—to conduct a detailed review of all relevant studies. The Institute of Medicine carefully examined all the studies that had been conducted on this subject and in 2004 concluded that there is no relationship between the MMR vaccine and autism.

In addition, most of the authors of the original study that incited the claim have changed their minds about their results. New data suggest that autism is caused much earlier, during fetal development, and that there may also be a genetic predisposition.

Similarly, the hepatitis B vaccine has been held responsible for several neurological disorders, such as multiple sclerosis and Guillain-Barré syndrome. However, studies have concluded that no data support these claims.

Some critics claim that the multiple vaccines administered during a child's early life can weaken, confuse, or misdirect the immune system, leading it either to overreact to antigens in the environment and thus cause asthma and allergies or to overreact to itself and cause autoimmune diseases. To many people, the current immunization schedule seems excessive—a baby can receive as many as fifteen injections during the first 6 months of his life. From a different perspective, however, the whole immunization schedule targets only fifteen germs. Imagine, in comparison, how many thousands of other microorganisms a child comes into contact with every day.

Young infants can respond to an estimated one hundred thousand different organisms at one time. Thus, vaccines do not "use up" all of the baby's immune system; in fact, they use only a minute portion of it. Moreover, today's vaccines are much purer than those of the past. All combined, the new vaccines contain fewer than two hundred proteins to stimulate antibody production compared with about three thousand proteins that used to be in the pertussis vaccine alone.

Many studies have shown no connection between multiple vaccines and a higher risk of infections, which would be expected from a weakened immune system. In fact, some vaccine-preventable viral infections, including measles and chickenpox, may themselves decrease the body's immunity for a while. Studies have also examined childhood diabetes and not found any links to multiple vaccines. To date, there are insufficient data to accept or reject a connection between multiple vaccines and the risk of asthma and allergies.

The last claim to mention is one that blamed vaccines for high mercury content. In the past, some vaccines did contain minute amounts of thimerosal, a mercury-containing preservative, which was added to vaccines to avoid bacterial or fungal contamination of vials used to administer multiple doses of a vaccine. The form of mercury in this preservative was ethyl mercury, which is different from either elemental mercury or methyl mercury. Both elemental mercury and methyl mercury can contaminate the environment and get into human foods, such as certain types of fish. These contaminants have been associated with neuropsychiatric disorders, including attention and speech disorders in children.

After carefully examining numerous studies and data on many thousands of children, the American Academy of Sciences concluded that the ethyl mercury in thimerosal contained in vaccines does not affect a child's neuropsychological development. Even so, the American Academy of Pediatrics recommended that all mercury be removed from vaccines, so most vaccines in use today for children do not contain mercury. The exceptions are some influenza vaccines and some meningococcal vaccine preparations that contain trace elements.

A factor that may have contributed to some of the erroneous beliefs about vaccine side effects was the establishment, in 1988, of a national compensation system for possible vaccine side effects. Called the National Vaccine Injury Compensation Program, this system was established to encourage the pharmaceutical industry to continue its efforts to produce new vaccines. The industry needed encouragement because of the numerous lawsuits they faced from individuals who believed that various serious conditions were the result of particular vaccines. The potential financial burden of these lawsuits threatened to bring the industry's vaccine work to a halt.

Therefore, the U.S. government removed the financial responsibility from the industry and undertook to compensate people if an illness started after a vaccine was administered, regardless of whether the vaccine was responsible for the condition. Receiving compensation did not necessarily mean that the vaccine caused the particular condition. However, the public has interpreted compensation to imply responsibility, thus contributing to many of the myths about some vaccine side effects. An additional reason for establishing this no-fault compensation system was to gather information and possibly identify previously unrecognized negative effects.

Scientific progress has made today's vaccines safer than ever before. And new research on genetic predisposition to side effects may help to prevent and avoid vaccine side effects in the future. If in doubt, look at what doctors do for their own children. Doctors are the most loyal supporters of vaccines, knowing full well the ramifications of not vaccinating, both for their children and for society. Indeed, compared with a century ago, humankind today is healthier, infant and child mortality are dramatically lower, and life expectancy is impressively longer. We owe these medical achievements primarily to vaccines, the miracle of infectious disease prevention.

Measures to Avoid Serious, Vaccine-Preventable Diseases

- Have your children vaccinated according to the recommended schedule to protect against many serious infectious diseases of infancy and childhood. These diseases used to claim many lives and cause serious illness in thousands of children.
- Keep serious diseases at bay by having your children vaccinated and by making sure you and your adolescent children receive appropriate booster doses.
- Know that despite the claims about many serious side effects, vaccines are very safe and serious side effects are extremely rare.
- Become informed about vaccines from reliable sources, like the American Academy of Pediatrics and the Centers for Disease Control and Prevention.
- Discuss all your questions with your doctor, including questions about vaccine use in children with preexisting medical conditions.

10

Baby's on the Way

PROTECT YOUR UNBORN BABY
WITH A HEALTHY PREGNANCY

Pregnancy should be a time for joy and anticipation as your baby grows within you and you look forward to the day when you finally meet your child face to face. As an expectant mother, you want to do everything you can for your baby to develop healthily. In addition to eating well, exercising appropriately, and getting enough sleep, you need to avoid contracting infections. Some infectious diseases carry risks for you as the expectant mother, but even more so, risks for your unborn baby. Unfortunately, some infections can have grave consequences for a developing fetus.

In this chapter, I discuss the main infections that can harm the fetus, and I provide information about preventing these infections. Many of the infections I mention in this chapter have already been discussed in earlier chapters, so in some cases, I refer you back to other chapters that may have additional information.

Infections That Can Affect the Developing Fetus

Any infection, particularly if it is serious, can negatively affect a pregnant woman's health, although in most cases, it is unlikely to threaten her life. For the fetus, however, infection is another story: some infections can severely affect the development and health or even the survival of the fetus. Serious illnesses during pregnancy can result in miscarriage, preterm birth, congenital anomalies (meaning defects present at birth), low birth weight, and other adverse consequences.

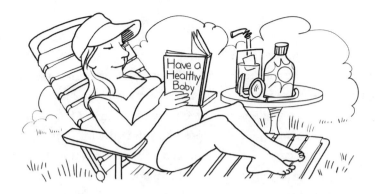

In some cases, an infection may not produce any symptoms in the baby until months or years after birth. For example, the baby or young child may develop vision problems from congenital toxoplasmosis; hearing problems from cytomegalovirus (CMV); vision, bone, and tooth abnormalities from syphilis; and immunosuppression from the AIDS virus.

In the United States, all newborns receive antibiotic eye drops against gonorrhea, regardless of whether the mother has the infection. In addition, any newborn (or baby 2 months or younger) who develops a fever should be checked by a pediatrician who may order blood, urine, or even spinal fluid tests. Very young infants are at higher risk of developing a bloodstream infection from the germs they encountered during the birth process or in their early surroundings.

The results of many studies provide a glimpse of the magnitude of congenital and neonatal infections in the United States: about 1 percent of all newborns have been infected with CMV, and shortly after birth, one to eight of every one thousand newborns become sick from a bacterial infection, usually derived from the mother. The immediate and long-term consequences of all such infections in children are a major problem worldwide.

There are three broad categories of infection that every pregnant woman should be aware of: sexually transmitted infections (STIs); infections that adults typically contract from children, among whom the illnesses primarily circulate; and infections transmitted from food, animals, or insect bites.

A woman can contract an STI before she gets pregnant or during her pregnancy, and she can transmit it to her baby at different times depending on the infection. Syphilis can cross the placenta and infect the fetus during pregnancy, while other infections, including chlamydia, gonorrhea, hepatitis B, and genital herpes can infect the baby as she passes through the birth canal. HIV can infect a baby both via the placenta and at birth, as well as through breast milk. In addition to causing a variety of problems and complications for the baby, which I discuss below for each infection, STIs can affect the pregnancy by causing the membranes around the baby to rupture early or by causing labor to begin early. The following discussion highlights the consequences of STIs for the fetus and infant; more details about the microbial causes and transmission of these infections are found in chapter 7.

Chlamydia is the most commonly reported STI in the United States—over 1.2 million cases were reported to the CDC in 2008. For a newborn, chlamydia can cause conjunctivitis (pink eye, an inflammation of the outer layer of the eye) and, less commonly, pneumonia. Chlamydia in a pregnant woman and in a baby can be treated with antibiotics.

Gonorrhea is also a common infection; the CDC estimates that in the United States, more than seven hundred thousand new cases of gonorrhea occur every year. A newborn who contracts gonorrhea during birth may get conjunctivitis (pink eye) or more severe eye infection. Rarely, a whole-body infection occurs. These complications in a newborn can be treated with antibiotics, as can gonorrhea in a pregnant woman.

Human papilloma viruses (HPVs), although extremely common, with the CDC estimating approximately 6 million new infections every year, are rarely transmitted to the newborn from the mother's genital tract. When transmission does occur, however, HPV can infect the baby's vocal cords, which can result in respiratory blockage.

According to the CDC, approximately one in five women ages 14 to 49 has genital herpes. This STI rarely infects the fetus during pregnancy, but it becomes very dangerous during the birth process. Infection with this virus in a newborn can cause eye infection, meningoencephalitis (infection of the brain and its coverings), or a general whole-body infection with very poor prognosis for mental development of the baby, if the baby even survives. For these reasons, a cesarean section is recommended if a woman has active herpes sores on the genitals when she is ready to give birth.

Group B *Streptococcus* is a sexually transmitted bacterium found in the genital tract or the intestine of the mother. Group B strep sometimes causes urinary tract infections in a pregnant woman, while at other times it does not cause any symptoms. About one-quarter of women carry the bacterium at some time. When the newborn comes into contact with this bacterium in the birth canal, she can contract the infection and become ill with meningitis, severe pneumonia, or a bloodstream infection. Because of these serious complications for the newborn, every pregnant woman should be checked for Group B strep toward the end of her pregnancy, and if she has the bacterium, she should be treated with antibiotics to prevent infection of the newborn. Typically, a woman who carries group B strep starts receiving antibiotics when she goes into labor, and the antibiotics continue to be administered throughout delivery.

Although less common today than it used to be, syphilis continues to exist; in 2006, nearly 350 babies were born in the United States with congenital syphilis. Syphilis can cause a multitude of abnormalities while the organs are forming in the fetus, and the damage can continue for several years after birth. It can damage the brain, eyes, bones, teeth, liver, and other organs. There is also a greater risk of an infected baby being stillborn or dying soon after birth. A baby born with congenital syphilis may not have any symptoms at birth, but if the disease goes untreated, the baby may become developmentally delayed, have seizures, or even die. Because of the severe consequences for the fetus, every pregnant woman should be checked for syphilis and treated with appropriate antibiotics if she becomes infected during pregnancy.

In 2007, an estimated forty-three thousand new hepatitis B infections occurred in the United States. There is a high rate of infection with the hepatitis B virus among babies born to infected mothers. In addition, when infected so young, infants have a 90 percent chance of developing chronic infection, which may progress to liver failure or liver cancer later in life. Hepatitis B is transmitted to the baby mainly at birth. Newborns of mothers with hepatitis B have to receive both the first dose of the hepatitis B vaccine and the specific immune globulin within the first twelve hours of life. The second vaccine dose is given at 1 to 2 months of age, and the third at 6 months. A hepatitis B-infected mother can breastfeed her baby, provided the baby has received the vaccine.

Hepatitis C can also be transmitted from mother to infant at the time of delivery. Unlike hepatitis B, however, the risk of transmission of hepatitis C from mother to infant is low, at less than 5 percent. Transmission of hepatitis C from breastfeeding has not been documented. Infected infants may develop chronic hepatitis and liver cirrhosis later in life.

Infection with the human immunodeficiency virus (HIV), which leads to AIDS, can be much better controlled in a pregnant woman today than a decade ago. The frequency of HIV transmission from mother to child has been reduced from 25 percent to less than 2 percent today thanks to combinations of antiviral drugs that can be taken during pregnancy. However, the key to decreasing the risk of HIV transmission to the baby is for combinations of antiretroviral medications to begin during early pregnancy and continue through labor and delivery. Therefore, it is very important that pregnant women be tested early in their pregnancy. If a pregnant woman has high levels of the virus in her blood despite receiving the medications, an elective cesarean section is recommended (before labor begins). The newborn should also receive medication for a period and be followed by a specialist, who will recommend appropriate testing to determine the baby's HIV status. An HIV-positive mother should not breastfeed her baby.

With all these precautions, the risk of HIV transmission from mother to baby is very low in the United States and in most developed countries (around 1 percent). Nevertheless, the CDC estimated that in 2005, 142 of the children newly diagnosed with HIV in the United States had contracted the virus from their mothers.

Infections Commonly Transmitted from Children

In the United States, cytomegalovirus (CMV) is the most common congenital infection, with about 1 percent of newborns infected by the virus. It is also the most common cause of noninherited deafness in children. About one-third to one-half of U.S. women of childbearing age have not been exposed to CMV, and therefore, they do not have antibodies against it.

If a pregnant woman without previous immunity contracts the virus, it can have harmful consequences for the fetus, causing damage to the brain, liver, or other organs and resulting in mental retardation, growth delay, or deafness. The risk of serious consequences to the fetus is highest during the first trimester of pregnancy. At birth, most infected newborns appear normal—only about 10 percent have symptoms—but they may later develop learning disabilities, mental retardation, or hearing problems. Pregnant women without immunity to CMV are most likely to contract the infection from toddlers, in whom CMV is quite frequent (and is unrelated to exposure in pregnancy).

Rubella, also known as German measles, is much less frequent today than in the past, because most women of childbearing age received the rubella vaccine as children. However, rubella does still occur in some women who have not received the vaccine or whose rubella antibodies have waned. Rubella during pregnancy can be devastating for the fetus, particularly if the mother contracts the infection during the first trimester of pregnancy. Rubella damages the fetus's brain, eyes, and heart. This congenital rubella syndrome is so devastating that if a pregnant woman without immunity contracts proven rubella during the first trimester of pregnancy, termination of the pregnancy will be recommended. All pregnant women should be checked for immunity (antibodies) to rubella.

Most U.S. women of childbearing age have immunity to chickenpox, because they had the infection during childhood. Some women escaped this common childhood illness, however, and are therefore susceptible as adults. Chickenpox in an adult is much more severe than in a child. If a susceptible pregnant woman is exposed to chickenpox, there is a small risk (about 2 to 3 percent) of the fetus developing abnormalities of the limbs (atrophy, or muscle wasting), the skin (scars), the brain, and the eyes. If exposed to the chickenpox virus, a susceptible pregnant woman should immediately receive the varicella immune globulin (not the vaccine). If a woman develops chickenpox a few days before or after delivery, the newborn should also receive the varicella immune globulin as soon as possible.

Parvovirus B19 causes a mild rash in children (fifth disease). In a pregnant woman, however, during the first half of pregnancy, this virus can infect the fetus and may result in a miscarriage. If the pregnancy continues, the fetus can develop anemia, which, if serious, may lead to body swelling and heart failure, though rarely. According to data from the CDC, about 50 percent of the population has not been previously exposed to parvovirus B19. If a pregnant woman is exposed to parvovirus B19, she should be checked for antibodies. If a susceptible woman is infected during her pregnancy, the fetus should be followed closely with repeated ultrasound exams of the heart. In severe cases, anemia can be managed with blood transfusions of the fetus inside the womb.

Enteroviruses, which mainly circulate during the summer months, cause a variety of symptoms, such as fever, rashes, cold symptoms, and even meningitis (usually mild). If a pregnant woman is infected near the end of her pregnancy, the newborn may become severely ill with meningitis, inflammation of the heart, or inflammation of the liver.

Influenza is serious for pregnant women, particularly in the third trimester, causing a higher risk for severe illness, complications, and hospitalization. The fetus is not directly affected by the flu, but serious illness in the mother could indirectly affect the fetus and cause preterm birth.

If you are exposed during your pregnancy to rubella, chickenpox, measles, hepatitis A, parvovirus B19, or any other childhood illness, you should talk to your doctor.

Infections Transmitted through Food, Animals, or Insects

Toxoplasmosis is a parasitic infection that, in children and adults, may have no symptoms whatsoever or only mild flulike symptoms, with fever and lymph node swelling. If this infection occurs during pregnancy, however, it can have serious consequences for the fetus, including mental retardation, inflammation of the liver, and vision problems. If a woman contracts the infection before getting pregnant, she will already have antibodies, and the risk of transmission to the fetus is much lower. The risk of fetal damage depends on when a woman is infected during pregnancy, with the risk highest during the first half and gradually decreasing throughout the pregnancy. A woman who contracts toxoplasmosis for the first time during pregnancy should receive appropriate antiparasitic therapy.

Listeriosis, a bacterial infection, produces flulike symptoms in a pregnant woman, such as fever, headache and muscle aches, and sometimes a mild diarrhea. In a newborn, it can cause a serious meningitis, pneumonia, or a severe bloodstream infection (septicemia); it can even induce preterm birth. This infection in newborns is treated with antibiotics.

Lymphocytic choriomeningitis is a viral infection that, in a newborn, causes a rare form of congenital infection, which is similar to that caused by CMV.

Finally, malaria is a threat for pregnant women traveling to malaria-endemic regions. Malarial infection in a pregnant woman is generally more severe than in a woman who is not pregnant. Consequences for the pregnancy can include miscarriage, premature delivery, and stillbirth.

How Can I Prevent Infections during My Pregnancy?

You can do much to prevent contracting an infection during your pregnancy. Some infections can be prevented with vaccines, so you should ensure that you have the necessary immunizations. In general, when you are pregnant, you should avoid contact with individuals with infectious diseases, particularly if you have not been exposed to the particular infection in the past. In addition, during your pregnancy, your doctor will check your urine for the presence of microorganisms. All urinary tract infections should be treated with appropriate antibiotics.

Sexually Transmitted Infections

Ideally, a woman should be tested for STIs before she becomes pregnant. Certainly, every pregnant woman should be checked during her pregnancy for some STIs: syphilis, group B streptococcus, hepatitis B, and HIV. She may be tested for other STIs depending on her individual risk for them. Hepatitis B can be prevented with a vaccine.

In some cases, a pregnant woman should take additional measures to prevent exposing her unborn baby to infection. For example, if a woman's sexual partner has herpes genital sores or is infected with HIV, the woman should avoid sexual contact throughout her pregnancy. Condoms should be used during pregnancy, because they decrease the risk of transmitting several STIs. I describe measures to protect against STIs in detail in chapter 7.

Infections Commonly Transmitted from Children

Many pregnant women have close contact with babies and toddlers, because they already have young children or they work at a day-care center, a preschool, or a children's hospital or clinic. All of these women, and particularly those who work with young children, are at higher risk of being exposed to CMV during their pregnancy. A pregnant woman who works with children older than 3 years of age has a lower risk of exposure to contaminated secretions. CMV is a highly contagious infection that is transmitted through contact with infected urine and saliva.

CMV is very common among young children, usually causing fever, cold symptoms, muscle aches, lymph node enlargement, and a mild inflammation of the liver. Children continue to excrete the virus for many months after their own symptoms have resolved, which is in part why women who work with young children are at such high risk of exposure. Studies in day-care centers in the United States have shown that as many as half of all children attending may excrete CMV in their saliva or urine at any particular time.

Ideally, pregnant women with high exposure to young children should be checked for antibodies against CMV before they become pregnant. A woman who is negative, meaning that she has never been infected with the virus and hasn't got antibodies, should be extremely careful to minimize her risk of exposure by thoroughly washing her hands after changing diapers and by avoiding exposure to toddlers' saliva. Studies have shown that pregnant women who practice heightened attention to hygiene (frequent hand washing, wearing gloves to change diapers, avoiding very close contact with toddlers, including kisses on the lips and on babies' hands) can lower their risk of exposure to CMV by up to 85 percent. In addition, a woman who tested negative to CMV antibodies and who works with young children might need to be checked for antibodies against the virus every month during the first half of her pregnancy.

A woman who is planning to become pregnant and knows or suspects that she has not received the rubella vaccine should be tested for antibodies. If she is negative for antibodies, she can be vaccinated and ideally will wait at least one month before becoming pregnant. Every woman is tested for rubella antibodies at the beginning of pregnancy. Likewise, a woman who has never had chickenpox and has not received the vaccine should be vaccinated prior to becoming pregnant (there are two vaccine doses, given one to two months apart) and, again, wait one month before conceiving.

The influenza vaccine (the injectable one) is recommended for all pregnant women whose second half of pregnancy will be during the fall and winter months. Getting the flu vaccine during pregnancy also protects the baby during the first months of her life, when she is too young to receive the flu vaccine or antiviral drugs. Pregnant women should always practice good hygiene, including frequent hand washing, to minimize the chances of contracting viruses such as parvovirus B19 and enteroviruses.

Infections Transmitted through Food, Animals, or Insects

Toxoplasmosis is transmitted through contact with cat feces and from eating meat that is inadequately cooked. It is more frequent in European countries (particularly in France) than in the United States, possibly because of the popularity of steak tartare, a dish made with raw beef. Other factors associated with an increased risk for toxoplasmosis include living in a neighborhood with a large number of stray cats, consuming raw vegetables and salads that have not been washed well (and that may have been in contact with cat feces), and consuming smoked pork and sausages. To avoid exposure to the *Toxoplasma* parasite, pregnant women should avoid eating raw or inadequately cooked lamb, pork, and beef. They should also avoid exposure to cat feces and objects that may have been contaminated by cats. In addition, pregnant women should wear gloves while gardening and wash their hands well after gardening activities.

Listeriosis, caused by the bacterium *Listeria monocytogenes*, is transmitted through unpasteurized cheeses, some pasteurized soft cheeses (for example, brie, camembert, ricotta), processed meat products, paté, and smoked and raw seafood. Pregnant women should pay particular attention to possible microbial contamination of their food and should avoid eating these foods.

Lymphocytic choriomeningitis is transmitted from the urine of mice, rats, hamsters, and other rodents. Pregnant women should avoid exposure to wild or pet rodents and their urine, feces, or other secretions.

Before traveling to a malaria-endemic region of the world, a woman who plans to become pregnant or who is already pregnant should take all necessary measures against contracting malaria. The ideal situation is to avoid traveling to regions with a high risk of malaria when pregnant, but if it is necessary, some malaria medications are safe to take during pregnancy. Chapter 6 has more information about malaria.

Can I Be Vaccinated while Pregnant?

Complete and regular immunization during childhood offers protection against vaccine-preventable diseases during a woman's reproductive years. However, some women have not received all recommended vaccines. As I discussed above, if you are not certain whether you are immune against rubella or chickenpox, you should be checked, ideally before pregnancy. If you do not have immunity, you should be vaccinated at least one month before getting pregnant.

In general, vaccines that contain dead or inactivated microorganisms, rather than live ones, are safe to have during pregnancy. Vaccines with dead or inactivated microorganisms are those against tetanus, diphtheria, pertussis, hepatitis B, and the injectable influenza vaccine. The influenza vaccine in particular is recommended for all pregnant women whose second half of pregnancy will be during flu season.

In contrast, vaccines that contain live attenuated microorganisms, such as those against measles, mumps, rubella, and chickenpox, as well as the nasally administered flu vaccine, should be avoided during pregnancy. If a pregnant woman already has a young child, the child can receive all recommended vaccinations as normal.

MAIN POINTS
Measures to Avoid Infections during Pregnancy

- Get vaccinated with all necessary vaccines before you become pregnant.
- Avoid vaccines containing live microorganisms during your pregnancy. These vaccines are the measles, mumps, rubella, and chickenpox vaccines and the nasally administered flu vaccine.

- Get vaccinated with the injectable flu vaccine during the fall or winter.
- When pregnant, get checked for sexually transmitted infections and follow your doctor's instructions about how to treat them.
- Avoid very close contact with babies and toddlers (such as kisses on the lips or hands and handling toys and objects that they bring to their mouth), and wash your hands carefully after changing diapers.
- Avoid cleaning cat litter boxes, and wear gloves when gardening.
- Avoid eating raw or inadequately cooked meat.
- Avoid eating unpasteurized dairy products and soft cheeses, even if they are pasteurized. Avoid eating paté; deli meats such as smoked sausages, prosciutto, and salami; and smoked salmon.
- Consult your doctor any time you are ill during your pregnancy (for example, if you have a fever, rash, or other symptoms, such as those of a urinary tract infection).

11

Bonding with Your Baby

THE BENEFITS OF BREASTFEEDING

One of the great joys for many new mothers is nursing their baby. For some women and their newborns, breastfeeding is as easy as putting baby to breast, the baby latches, and the milk flows. For other women and newborns, the art of breastfeeding takes practice and perseverance. The perseverance is worth it, though. Beyond breast milk's nutritional value and the maternal-infant bond that it strengthens, it contains substances that strengthen a baby's defenses against germs.

The American Academy of Pediatrics recommends that U.S. women continue breastfeeding for their baby's first year of life, or even longer, if the mother and baby mutually wish it. In addition, the World Health Organization recommends breastfeeding for resource-limited countries without adequate sanitation and clean water supply. In these countries, breastfeeding is estimated to save the lives of more than 1 million children annually, children who would otherwise succumb to respiratory and gastrointestinal infections.

At six months, babies begin to eat solids and other foods, but breast milk should continue to be part of their diet. If you can, there is no harm, only benefit, to continuing to breastfeed even longer than a year. Breastfeeding is a personal decision, of course, and some women choose not to breastfeed for various reasons. From a medical point of view, however, there are only a few instances, such as when a mother is infected with HIV, when a woman should not breastfeed her baby. Many of the reasons for which women believe they should stop breastfeeding, such as having a cold, are not in fact a problem for continuing to nurse.

In this chapter, I discuss whether or not breastfeeding can continue uninterrupted when a nursing mother has an infection, gets a vaccine, or takes antibiotics. First, though, I describe the benefits of breast milk for a baby's immune system.

Why Is Breast Milk So Good for Babies?

Breast milk is designed to be a baby's complete diet in his first six months of life. An excellent source of nutrition, it is rich in essential amino acids, proteins, carbohydrates, and fats. A breastfed baby does not need anything else, not even water, in these first few months of life. In addition to covering all of a baby's nutritional needs, breast milk has unique properties that are impossible for formulas to accurately copy. Breast milk's composition changes as a baby grows, so breast milk is truly tailored to the baby's needs.

Breast milk contains all kinds of antibodies. In particular, it has immunoglobulin A, or IgA, antibodies, which are found only in secretions. These antibodies are produced in the breast either by cells that migrate to the breast from the mother's intestine or by cells in the breast that receive a signal from intestinal cells to produce the antibodies. The IgA antibodies that result from this enteromammary, or intestine-to-breast, cycle, confer potent protection to a baby against germs that his mother has encountered in the past and which he is also likely to encounter. These antibodies are not found in formulas that derive from cow's milk.

In addition, a breastfed baby gets antibodies that circulate in the mother's blood, such as antibodies against vaccine-preventable diseases like tetanus and the flu. Therefore, if the mother has been vaccinated, the baby is also protected in the first few months of life. These antibodies are IgG antibodies found in the blood and pass into the breast milk.

Breast milk also includes other substances with antimicrobial action, such as lysozyme, lactoferrin, casein, and many others. These substances help babies fight infection. Last, breast milk contains probiotics, which are live bacteria that have benefits for health. I discuss probiotics in chapter 12.

Given these ingredients, it is not surprising that babies who are breastfed for at least three months have half the incidence of gastrointestinal

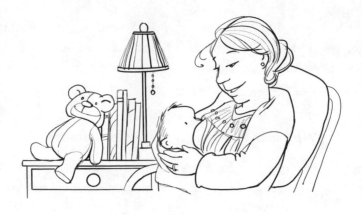

infections. They also have fewer respiratory, ear, and lung infections such as bronchiolitis, which may lead to childhood asthma. As well as reducing the number of infections, breast milk lowers the duration and severity of infections in breastfed children compared with formula-fed children. The benefits are greater if the baby has been exclusively breastfed for at least three months.

There are indications that other, more serious infections, including urinary tract infections, sepsis, and necrotizing enterocolitis—the latter two being life-threatening conditions, particularly for premature babies— are less frequent and less severe in breastfed babies. Breastfeeding also protects a baby from developing asthma, allergies, diabetes, obesity, and some cancers (leukemias), and there is some evidence that breastfeeding may increase a child's intelligence scores.

There is one nutrient that breastfed babies do not receive in sufficient quantity from breast milk. Vitamin D is present only in low levels, so all full-term infants who are breastfed should be given a supplement of 400 IU of vitamin D per day.

Common Questions about Breastfeeding and Infection

Can I Be Vaccinated while Nursing?

Yes, you can. Vaccines are safe while you are nursing, even vaccines that contain live viruses. No data indicate that live viruses in vaccines can harm a baby through breast milk. The only vaccine virus that has been found to pass into a mother's milk is the rubella virus, but it will not harm the baby.

Nursing mothers can receive the following vaccines without any problem: measles, mumps, rubella, tetanus, diphtheria, influenza, *Pneumococcus*, hepatitis A, hepatitis B, and chickenpox. A nursing mother who has not been immunized against polio and has to travel to a polio-endemic area of the world should receive the injectable polio vaccine. Also, a breastfed baby can receive all recommended vaccines as normal.

Can I Nurse if I Have an Infection?

Yes, in most cases. If you contract a viral infection such as a cold, the flu, or gastroenteritis, or a bacterial infection like staph infections of the skin or urinary tract infections, you can and should continue nursing.

Even with symptoms of mastitis—a breast infection that causes swelling, redness, and pain, usually in one breast—a nursing mother can continue to breastfeed her baby. Mastitis results from a blocked milk duct that is then colonized by bacteria, but even though these bacteria can pass into breast milk, most healthy babies are not put at risk by them. If your baby is premature or has other medical problems, your pediatrician will advise you about the safety of continuing to nurse with mastitis. A woman with mastitis needs to take antibiotics and must continue to remove the milk from her breast either by pumping or by nursing. The antibiotics may get into the breast milk, but most antibiotics do not cause a problem for the baby (more on antibiotics in a moment).

If, rarely, a breast abscess (a collection of pus in the breast) develops, a nursing mother should stop breastfeeding temporarily from the affected breast, until the infection is treated appropriately, but she should continue to remove milk by pumping her breasts so that milk production does not stop. Your doctor will advise you when to stop breastfeeding if you have a breast infection.

A few other infections are not a problem for most babies:

- Cytomegalovirus (CMV) passes into breast milk but does not pose a problem for a healthy baby unless he is premature. In this case, your pediatrician will guide you according to your specific circumstances and what is best for your baby.

- A mother with hepatitis B can nurse her baby provided the baby received the hepatitis B vaccine and immune globulin on the first day of his life. He must also have the subsequent booster doses at 1 to 2 months and 6 months.
- A mother with hepatitis C can nurse her baby. Although transmission of this virus to the baby through breastfeeding is theoretically possible, it has never been shown to occur.

Some infections *can* be a problem for a baby:

- In the United States, Europe, and other countries with a safe water supply, a mother with HIV infection should not nurse her baby, because HIV can be transmitted to the baby in the breast milk.
- A mother with a herpes sore on the breast should avoid breastfeeding until the sore is healed.
- A mother with active tuberculosis that has not been treated should not nurse or have other close contact with her baby until she starts appropriate therapy and is no longer contagious.
- A mother who develops chickenpox five days before through two days after delivery should be separated from her baby, but her milk can be expressed and used for feeding.
- A mother with H1N1 influenza should be separated from her newborn until her fever is gone. She can still express milk for feeding.

Can I Continue Nursing while on Antibiotics or Other Medications?

It depends on the antibiotic or medication. If you are nursing and you have to take antibiotics or other medications, always ask your obstetrician's and pediatrician's advice, because many medications pass into breast milk and from the milk to the baby.

Most antibiotics do not cause any problems for a baby, but there are some notable exceptions. For this reason, you should always mention that you are nursing so the physician prescribing a medication for you can determine if it is safe or if another one might be preferable. In addition, ask your doctor about the safety for your breastfed baby of all medications that you take, including over-the-counter medications, herbs, and food supplements.

How Can I Safely Preserve Breast Milk?

If you want to preserve your milk to feed your baby at a later time or to have someone else feed your baby, put the freshly pumped milk in a clean container and refrigerate it immediately. Use the milk within twenty-four hours.

Breast milk can be kept in the freezer for about three months. When you remove frozen milk from the freezer, let it thaw in the refrigerator or in a bowl of warm water for immediate use. Never defrost breast milk in the microwave, because it may destroy some of the milk's components.

In some circumstances, such as when a mother does not have her own milk supply, babies born prematurely may be fed milk that is collected from donors. Many donor milk banks belong to the Human Milk Banking Association of North America and follow guidelines to screen the milk for a number of infectious microorganisms, such as HIV, hepatitis B and C, HTLV 1 and 2 (human T-lymphotropic viruses), and syphilis. Donor milk is also heat treated (pasteurized) to destroy any bacteria or HIV that may be present. Heat treatment may also affect some nutrients and bioactive factors in breast milk, so whenever possible, fresh milk from the mother herself is preferable for feeding an infant.

⊢ MAIN POINTS ⊢
Measures to Give Your Baby the Benefits of Breast Milk

- If possible, breastfeed your baby to give him the ideal nutrition of breast milk along with its multiple other benefits, such as immune factors that protect him from infections.
- Always ask your doctor whether antibiotics or other medications you may take are safe for your breastfed baby.
- Be reassured that it is safe to continue breastfeeding through most minor maternal infections.
- Know that vaccines are safe for mother and baby during breast-feeding, and they can be administered as normal.

Supplements, Herbs, Organic Produce, and Probiotics

DO THEY PROTECT YOU FROM GERMS?

Every day, news stories, articles, and advertisements bombard us with information about our health—or lack of health—and what we can do or take to improve it. The number and variety of available food supplements and herbs are truly astounding and, for many people, completely confusing. In addition, at grocery stores, we now have the choice of buying some fruits, vegetables, meats, and dairy products produced either with conventional farming methods or with organic farming methods. For many consumers, the true differences between the two remain mysterious, although the difference in the price tag is usually clear. Probiotics also appear on product labels these days, on foods like yogurt and in some beverages and supplements. In this chapter, I discuss these four types of products—food supplements, herbs, organic foods, and probiotics—in terms of their ability to boost your children's immune system and protect them from germs.

Daily Nutrition:
Does Your Child Need Food Supplements?

Parents want their children to be healthy, and most realize that diet is a critical factor. Frequently, however, parents wonder whether their children get all the nutrition their growing bodies need and whether they ought to take supplements of one kind or another. In studies performed

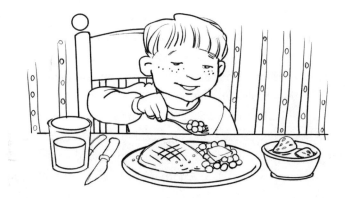

among poor, undernourished populations of Central America, supplemental food given to pregnant women and toddlers had a positive effect. There were 20 percent fewer fatalities in infants and young children who contracted diarrhea or respiratory infections, two common causes of death in children in developing countries.

But are food supplements necessary for most children in the United States? Most important for the proper functioning and development of a child's body is a varied and balanced diet. Beyond its other benefits, a balanced diet bolsters the immune system and assures that the body's defenses are ready to act against microbial hazards in the environment. Any stressful factor, such as a serious infection or other illness, increases the body's nutritional needs, so your children must consume adequate amounts of proteins, vitamins, and trace elements. These dietary needs are best met by eating food, however, not by taking supplements.

In addition, most supplements do not undergo rigorous clinical testing and are not subject to the strict regulations that medications undergo, so often there is no guarantee that a product's contents are indeed the same as what is written on the package label.

Amino Acids

Amino acids are the building blocks of proteins. Proteins are an essential part of a child's diet, because they are necessary for all metabolic functions, including the formation of antibodies (in fact, antibodies are proteins) and other important components of the immune system. It is proved and widely recognized that the best source of protein for newborns and older babies is breast milk. The makers of infant formulas have devoted years of research in their effort to mimic the components of breast milk. After infancy, good sources of protein are meat, dairy products, and some vegetables and legumes.

In clinical studies, some amino acids, such as glutamine and arginine, have proved beneficial in lowering the number of serious infections contracted by premature babies, intensive care patients, patients with severe burns, and patients with AIDS. Another study showed that glutamine supplements lowered the number of viral and other infections in marathon runners. No data suggest, however, that amino acid supplements are necessary in healthy individuals who are not exposed to extreme biological stress.

Children do not need amino acid supplements. A diet that includes poultry, meat, fish, vegetables, beans, and dairy is rich in amino acids. Moreover, there is no risk of side effects from eating these foods, while commercially available amino acid supplements may have risks of side effects along with their doubtful benefit.

Vitamins

The term "vitamins" includes more than twelve substances that are necessary for various vital body functions. Specific disorders develop as a result of the body not having enough of a particular vitamin. For example, a deficiency of vitamin C can cause scurvy, and a deficiency of vitamin D can cause rickets. Conversely, excessively high levels of some vitamins are also dangerous. For example, vitamin A overdose can cause toxicity, with problems for the brain, liver, skin, and hair. The human body cannot synthesize most vitamins, so we must get them from our diet. A variety of foods contain vitamins.

Your pediatrician may recommend that your child take vitamins for many reasons, but to bolster the immune system in order to prevent infections, vitamin supplements are rarely necessary. A full and balanced diet offers sufficient quantities of all vitamins needed by the body. Here, I discuss the results of clinical studies that have examined the insufficiency of particular vitamins and the effects of supplementing with these vitamins on susceptibility to infections.

Vitamin A (and beta-carotene, which is converted into vitamin A in the body) is involved in defending the body against microbes. In countries with insufficient food supply, such as many African countries, vitamin A supplements given to children ages 6 months to 5 years lowered their risk of death by up to 30 percent. In particular, fewer children died from measles and diarrhea, both frequent causes of death in undernourished children. In contrast, vitamin A had no effect in these children on the risk of severe pneumonia, another frequent cause of childhood death. In countries with adequate food supply and nutrition, however, studies have not shown a benefit of vitamin A supplements in healthy children and adults who consume a good diet. In fact, giving high doses of vitamin A can cause serious problems. Vitamin A supplements are not necessary for children who eat a full and balanced diet.

Vitamin C gained popularity in 1970 when the Nobel Prize laureate Linus Pauling published a monograph about its beneficial effects in preventing and treating the common cold. Since then, many studies have examined the purported effects of large doses of vitamin C. Overall, the results do not support vitamin C as a beneficial treatment when someone has already become sick with the common cold. Studies that examined whether vitamin C has a role in *preventing* the common cold, however, yielded more encouraging results. Individuals who took vitamin C supplements developed the same number of colds as people who did not take the supplements, but the duration and severity of their colds were slightly lower.

Does this mean that you should give your children vitamin C every day? Yes, absolutely: through their diet. Many foods, including fruits and vegetables, contain vitamin C. Some experts recommend taking vitamin C supplements (250 mg per day) when somebody else in the household is sick with a cold. In these cases, a child is at much higher risk of contracting the virus. Thus, rather than giving your child daily vitamin C supplements in an attempt to prevent a few of the six to ten upper respiratory infections that she will have, on average, each year, save the supplements to give to her only when another family member has cold symptoms. The rest of the time, encourage her to eat fresh vegetables and fruits, including orange juice. The vitamin C in these foods is enough.

Vitamin D has sparked a lot of interest lately, because vitamin D deficiency has been associated with many ill effects, including osteoporosis, bone fractures, cancer, diabetes, and immune system dysfunction. Vitamin D is formed in the body when the skin is exposed to sunlight, particularly ultraviolet sunrays. A recent study showed that dark skin does not absorb ultraviolet sunrays very well, and people with dark skin do not produce sufficient levels of some of the immune factors that fight the tuberculosis mycobacterium. Other recent studies have shown that many adolescents in the United States have low levels of vitamin D from inadequate exposure to the sun. Factors associated with inadequate exposure included living in the northeastern states, being obese, and not getting enough physical activity.

Some evidence may link vitamin D insufficiency to seasonal flu and respiratory infections, like the common cold. One study connected the body's lower levels of vitamin D during winter, when we have less exposure to sunlight, with the higher frequency of colds at this time of year. Certainly, other factors play a role in wintertime colds, too, including greater crowding, school schedules, and changes in germ contagiousness at different temperatures. Another study, which examined more than eighteen thousand Americans ages 12 and older, found that people with the lowest levels of vitamin D in their body were 36 percent more likely to have had a respiratory infection compared with people with the highest vitamin D levels.

The American Academy of Pediatrics (AAP) has doubled the amount of vitamin D it recommends for infants, children, and adolescents to 400 International Units (IU) per day. Breast milk does not contain sufficient vitamin D, so a breastfed newborn should be given vitamin D supplements starting in the first few days of life. The supplements should be continued until a baby gets enough vitamin D from her diet, which is achieved if she is weaned to vitamin D–fortified formula or vitamin D–fortified milk. (A baby who is not drinking breast milk should drink infant formula until at least age 1, and only at this age can she begin to drink cow's milk.)

Children should get enough vitamin D from milk and dairy products if they drink at least one quart of milk per day. Exposure to sunlight helps, too, although because of the higher risk of skin cancer in later life, the

AAP recommends that infants and young children not be exposed to direct sunlight outside, and that all children use sunscreen when in the sun. Because the sunscreen prevents vitamin D from being formed in the skin, children must take enough vitamin D through their diet, with supplements if milk products are restricted in the diet.

Adolescents who do not consume 400 IU of vitamin D per day through foods, because they are vegan or have otherwise restricted diets, or who do not have adequate exposure to the sun (which is difficult to measure) should also take a supplement containing this amount. The vitamin D story will undoubtedly evolve, so stay tuned.

Trace Elements

Trace elements are mainly minerals that the body needs in minute quantities. Children who eat a balanced diet get all the trace elements they need. Many people believe that some elements, such as zinc and selenium, help the immune system and prevent colds and other infections. In developing countries with malnutrition problems, zinc supplements have indeed been found to decrease the number of respiratory and diarrheal infections in babies and young children. However, the results of clinical studies examining the role of zinc in preventing colds in the United States and other developed countries are controversial. The data available to date are insufficient to justify giving zinc supplements to healthy children who eat a balanced diet, and the use of these supplements can have side effects. For example, intranasal formulations of zinc, marketed to prevent the common cold, were recently recalled in the United States because in several cases, they caused anosmia, which is the inability to smell.

From Garlic to Ginseng: Do Herbs Strengthen the Immune System?

Herbs are certain plants used for various purposes, including culinary and medicinal ones. Herbs and pharmaceuticals share a common history. Many of our most important medications, from aspirin to atropine, are derived from plants. And most of us consume at least one herbal concoction every day: coffee or tea. On the other hand, some herbal extracts are known to have harmful effects for our health, tobacco being a prime example. In addition to these more familiar herbs, many other herbal products are sold in the form of tablets, capsules, or solutions as alternative treatments for a multitude of illnesses or as supplements to prevent illnesses.

Many people claim that some herbs and other plants, such as *Echinacea, Andrographis*, ginseng, and garlic have beneficial properties that strengthen the immune system and lower the risk of contracting colds and other infections. There is no proof, however, from independent clinical studies—that is, studies not sponsored by product manufacturers—that any of these substances can indeed prevent colds in children. Clinical studies of garlic have found a slight benefit in lowering cholesterol and high blood pressure, but no antimicrobial effect has been proved. Studies have found that chamomile has beneficial effects as a mild relaxant and for wound healing.

On the other hand, several herbs can have side effects. For example, *Echinacea* can often cause a rash, itchiness, headache, and stomachache, and *Andrographis* has been reported to cause severe allergic reactions, headache, swollen lymph glands, nausea, diarrhea, and a metallic taste. Even if an herb has proven clinical safety and effectiveness, there are no guarantees about the quality of a particular product containing that herb, because these products do not undergo the same rigorous clinical testing as pharmaceuticals. Therefore, you cannot be sure that a product contains what its packaging claims, particularly for more expensive herbs like ginseng. In some cases, products marketed as ginseng have been analyzed to find that ginseng was completely absent.

In addition, herbal products often contain heavy metals, pesticides, or other herbs or pharmaceuticals. A recent study of Ayurvedic herbal products, half of which were marketed for children, found that 20 percent contained heavy metals such as lead, arsenic, or mercury. A study of herbal remedies imported from China showed that 30 percent of the products contained substances other than those listed on the package, including potent pharmaceuticals like phenacetin and steroids. In addition, many herbs and plant derivatives may interact with other medications.

In short, do not give your children herbal supplements.

To Buy or Not to Buy:
Should You Give Your Child Organic Foods?

The organic foods movement has increased significantly in the last several years. The Organic Trade Association reports that in 2009, U.S. sales of organic foods and beverages totaled $24.8 billion, approximately 4 percent of overall food and beverage sales that year—the industry is not insignificant. Today, most grocery stores sell at least a few foods that are labeled as organic.

Organic foods are popular among consumers keen to avoid pesticides, synthetic fertilizers, industrial waste, preservatives, and, in the case of meat products, hormones and antibiotics. Many people worry that chronic exposure to these chemicals has harmful health effects. Indeed, health problems, including fetal abnormalities, neurological disorders, fertility problems, immune system disorders, and cancer, have been observed in experimental animals exposed to large doses of such chemicals for long periods. The doses that people are exposed to in food are much lower than the doses in the experimental animal studies, and we do not know how the results translate for human health over a lifetime.

Farmers who use organophosphate pesticides, and are therefore exposed to high concentrations when applying them, have developed health problems, including a higher incidence of neurological disorders and cancers. Organophosphate levels in foods are very low by the time the products are harvested and sold. Nevertheless, they can be detected in foods, even in commercial baby foods.

A recent study indicated that consuming organic produce is associated with a lower risk of food-borne infections. However, this finding needs to be confirmed with additional research before it can be accepted as a fact. People clearly can acquire bacteria, such as *E. coli* and others, that are resistant to antibiotics, from eating meat and poultry that have been fed antibiotics. Most non-organically raised animals have been given antibiotics to stimulate their growth. As I discussed in chapter 8, antibiotic-resistant bacteria are hazardous for human health.

Some researchers have claimed that organic produce contains higher concentrations of some antioxidants, vitamins, and trace elements and is therefore more nutritious than non-organic produce. Again, these claims require more research. Conventionally grown produce is a nutritious source of many dietary needs. Even though it is more expensive to buy, organic produce cannot be kept fresh as long as conventional produce, not having been exposed to pesticides and antibiotics that prevent the growth of bacteria, fungi, and insects. (See the box about irradiation as a technique to sterilize and preserve foods.)

In the United States, Canada, the European Union, Japan, and other countries, rules and regulations govern the production and labeling of foods sold as organic. Organic food producers need to comply with specific restrictions during farming and production. In most cases, however, certain chemicals and pesticides are indeed allowed in organic production. Of course, hormones, antibiotics, synthetic dyes, and preservatives are not used on organic produce to boost its growth or to make it more presentable for sale, so consuming organic produce will prevent exposure to most of these chemicals.

When you are food shopping, keep in mind a few things as you decide whether to select organic versus conventional foods:

- Regulations governing organic food production are not uniform everywhere, and they may not always be enforced. Foods labeled as organic might differ depending on where the food is produced. Always carefully read the product label.
- Organic vegetables and fruits, even when cultivated without synthetic fertilizers, as you may do in your garden, can still contain low levels of chemicals from the soil, air, and rainwater.
- Organic vegetables are also at risk of being contaminated with microbes, because some organic manure is not sterilized and can contain harmful germs.
- In general, the fruits and vegetables with the highest levels of pesticides are apples, pears, cherries, peaches, strawberries, potatoes, peppers, and spinach.
- The fruits and vegetables that concentrate much lower levels of pesticides in their flesh are bananas, pineapple, broccoli, asparagus, corn, onions, peas, and cauliflower. The Environmental Working Group rates fruits and vegetables on their website, www.foodnews.org/walletguide.php.

Food Irradiation

Approximately forty countries have approved food irradiation, which uses small doses of ionizing radiation to sterilize food from harmful bacteria such as *E. coli* and *Salmonella*. Irradiation also destroys fungi, insects, and parasites. In addition, irradiation slows down the ripening process, and slows down rotting in foods like potatoes, onions, garlic, and others. Many experts believe that irradiation is the safest method of food preservation, safer than many of the additives and other preservatives in current use. Contrary to the fears of many consumers, irradiation does not make the food radioactive.

Critics claim that during irradiation new chemicals form, such as cyclo-butanones, and these may have harmful effects on health over the long term. To date, scientific studies with sufficiently long follow-up have not been done to prove or disprove these claims, so it is still too early to know.

According to the U.S. Food and Drug Administration, food irradiation may lead to a small loss of nutritional elements, but no more than from other food handling methods, such as cooking, pasteurizing, and canning. In the United States, food irradiation is currently used for flour, potatoes, eggs, meats, spices, and several kinds of fresh produce. In all cases, the package label must state that the food has been irradiated.

Good Bacteria: How Can Probiotics Help Your Child?

Probiotics are live microorganisms that have beneficial effects for our health. They include the so-called good bacteria that exist in the body to help with food digestion, produce antimicrobial peptides (called *defensins*), and protect against the bad, or pathogenic, bacteria. There are also substances called *prebiotics*, which do not contain microorganisms but which promote the growth and replication of good bacteria in the body. Examples of prebiotics include fructo-oligosaccharides and galacto-oligosaccharides, which are non-absorbable hydrocarbons.

Probiotics may be consumed by eating or drinking foods that natu-rally contain probiotic microorganisms or by eating or drinking foods that have been supplemented with probiotics. Probiotics may also be taken as a supplement in pill, capsule, or powder form. We all have good bacteria in our intestinal tract, so the idea of eating foods containing probiotics is that they will add to the number of good bacteria in the body. The most widely known and available probiotic food is yogurt, which contains *Lactobacillus* and other microorganisms. Other products containing probiotics, such as *Lactobacillus rhamnosus* GG, *Lactobacillus acidophilus*, and *Bifidobacterium*, either individually or as mixed cultures, include enriched yogurts, milk, juices, liquid fermented dairy products, and supplements. These enriched products are sometimes called *Lactobacillus* preparations. Prebiotics are usually nondigestible fibers, and they occur naturally in many foods like artichokes, berries, bananas, leafy greens, onions, legumes, and grains. Some foods are also fortified with them, including some yogurts, drinks, and energy bars. Human breast milk contains both prebiotic substances and probiotic bacteria.

Eating probiotic-containing foods to introduce good bacteria into the body may alter the composition of microorganisms in the intestine, but usually only temporarily because, in a sense, the body knows its natural microbes. Beyond infancy, efforts to change or add to the bacteria in the intestine may cause an immune reaction against the new microorganisms, and the body will eliminate them from the intestinal tract in many cases. The body reacts this way because of how the immune system develops early in life. During the birth process, a baby is exposed to germs for the first time, and over the first months of life, the immune system learns to recognize the bacteria present at that time as good ones. Therefore, microorganisms swallowed soon after birth are well tolerated for a person's whole life and make up the intestine's natural microbial community.

The microbial composition of a baby's intestine depends on factors like how she was born (vaginally or by cesarean section) and her diet (breast milk or formula). Babies born vaginally are exposed to more of their mothers' germs, and may have a lower incidence of allergic problems later in life. In addition, breastfed babies have more of the good germ *Bifidobacterium* in their intestine and also may have a lower incidence of allergic problems later in life. Of course, breast milk contains multiple other immune factors, and deciphering the role each factor plays is not an easy task.

The observations that vaginally born and breastfed babies are less likely to develop allergies may be connected to the hygiene hypothesis, which was proposed in 1989 and purports that infections during early infancy may protect a child from future allergies. (I discuss the hygiene hypothesis in chapter 13.) Other researchers have proposed that the initial microbial composition in the gut is an important factor in whether a child later develops allergies or autoimmune disorders. Recent findings indicate that the story is more complex; for example, genetic factors also seem to affect the composition of the microbial flora in the gut.

Probiotics are thought to interact with the microorganisms naturally found in the intestine, as well as with the mucosal membranes and the immune cells in the gut. Through these interactions, probiotics may affect the immune responses of the intestinal tract, decrease local inflammation, strengthen the defenses against pathogenic bacteria, and decrease the body's reaction against itself (as happens with autoimmune disorders).

Probiotics have been used to reduce the symptoms of a wide range of illnesses. In general, clinical studies have shown that probiotics have a benefit in treating viral diarrheas, antibiotic-related diarrhea, traveler's diarrhea, eczema, and irritable colon syndrome. Preliminary data also indicate that probiotics may benefit people with conditions such as lactose intolerance, high blood cholesterol, dental plaque, respiratory infections, rheumatoid arthritis, Crohn's disease, diabetes, colon cancer, and infant allergies and asthma.

Many children (and adults) develop diarrhea when they take antibiotics to treat an infection, because antibiotics kill not only the harmful bacteria in the gut but also the good ones. Sometimes, taking antibiotics leads to the bacterium *C. difficile* taking over in the intestinal tract and producing a toxin that leads to bloody diarrhea. Studies have shown that consuming probiotics during and following a course of antibiotics may decrease the risk of antibiotic-related diarrhea. Other studies have shown that probiotics decrease the duration of diarrhea caused by bacterial or viral gastroenteritis. Studies that examined probiotics for a role in preventing diarrhea, however, have been less convincing. Some studies have indicated that probiotics can prevent traveler's diarrhea, but others have not found this benefit.

I recommend that your child eat probiotic-containing yogurt every day when she is taking antibiotics, both during the antibiotic course and for several days afterward. In addition, give your child yogurt if she has diarrhea, because the probiotics may decrease its duration by a day or more. *Lactobacillus* and other probiotic preparations have an effect similar to yogurt.

Some other infections may be prevented or ameliorated if you eat foods containing probiotics, but on the whole, study results are not yet conclusive. Probiotics may or may not help to prevent vaginal yeast infections in women who get them frequently. It certainly will not hurt, though, to add yogurt to your daughter's diet if she has a vaginal yeast infection. (Of course, she should also receive proper treatment for the infection.) Although not related to probiotics, fresh acidic juices, particularly cranberry juice, might help prevent urinary tract infections in girls, because they make the urine and the bladder less hospitable to bacteria; not all studies have confirmed this piece of folk wisdom, however.

Respiratory infections may or may not be affected by probiotics. A clinical study found a 20 percent decrease in the incidence of bronchitis, ear infections, and pneumonia when probiotic-enriched milk was given to children attending day care. However, this study has not been confirmed by others. Last, the finding that *Lactobacillus* can prevent the formation of dental plaque in children ages 3 to 4 years can be considered only preliminary at this point.

Some recently developed infant formulas now have probiotic preparations added to them. The theory behind these new formulas is that breast-fed babies have more of the good germs, like *Bifidobacterium*, in their intestinal tract and a lower incidence of infections compared with formula-fed babies. The studies to date, however, have not been convincing in showing that probiotic-enriched formulas offer a real benefit to babies, and not enough is known about possible side effects. For premature babies studies have shown that there is a benefit from probiotic-enriched formula in decreasing both the chance and the seriousness of necrotizing enterocolitis, a life-threatening disease. However, given a premature baby's immature immune system, the safety of giving live microorganisms needs to be further evaluated before general recommendations are made for the use of such formulas.

The future of probiotics could be an interesting one. Some bold, visionary scientists have imagined the future possibility of "taming" germs and using them in the environment for health benefits. These scientists believe that in the future a cocktail of probiotics could be used as soaps and cleaning products on our skin and on objects in our environment. The aim would be not to sterilize objects and our skin but to colonize them with beneficial bacteria. Right now, this vision may sound like science fiction, but it does have some theoretical advantages. We will have to wait and see what the future holds.

─────────────────┤ MAIN POINTS ├─────────────────
Dietary Measures to Avoid Infections

- Make sure that your children eat a full and balanced diet.
- Don't give food supplements to children who eat a balanced diet, because supplements are not necessary to prevent or treat infections.
- Babies exclusively breastfed need vitamin D supplements, as do children who consume vegan diets and children who consume less than about a quart of milk or other dairy products per day.
- Avoid herbal products in children, because many of them may have side effects and their benefit is not proved.
- Know that true organic foods minimize exposure to hormones, pesticides, and antibiotics, but they have no proven benefit for the immune system's function.
- Eat foods containing probiotics (such as yogurt), because they help to treat viral and bacterial diarrheas, as well as antibiotic-related diarrhea, and they may help to prevent some diarrheas too.

13

Wash Your Hands!

PERSONAL AND HOUSEHOLD HYGIENE
FOR THE TWENTY-FIRST CENTURY

Given what we know today about germs, it seems extraordinary that until the mid-1800s, doctors did not wash their hands between patients or operations. We owe the practice of hand washing to Ignaz Semmelweis, a Hungarian obstetrician. In his day, many women who had just delivered a baby would become ill and die from serious infection. Semmelweis, working at the Vienna General Hospital, noticed in 1846 that a common factor in infections right after delivery was an obstetrician who had performed an autopsy before assisting at the delivery. He thought that the doctor might have carried "particles" on his hands from the cadaver to the woman.

When Semmelweis asked obstetricians at the hospital to wash their hands with a bleach solution after autopsies and before deliveries, the frequency of infections in new mothers decreased markedly. Thus, medical and hospital hygiene—considered basic 150 years later—was born. (However, the medical establishment during Semmelweis' tenure ignored and rejected his theory, and Semmelweis died in a psychiatric asylum. His recommended hand-sanitizing practice became widely accepted many years after his death, after Pasteur developed the microbial theory, also known as the germ theory of disease, in the mid-1860s.)

In earlier chapters, I've mentioned several important elements of hygiene, including the habits we, as parents, should both practice and instill in our children when at home, at school, outdoors, playing sports, and around pets. I have also described household cleaning practices that help to prevent food-borne illnesses and other infections.

In this chapter, I summarize the most important components of hygiene and take a microbiological "tour" through the rooms of a house. I describe the basic hygiene rules that we learned from our mothers—the most important one being good hand washing—and talk about some new dimensions of hygiene, such as using antibacterial soap and cleaning products. Last, I discuss the hygiene hypothesis, a recent theory proposing that excessive cleaning of a child's environment may increase his chances of developing allergic and autoimmune disorders in later life. Is cleanliness dangerous? Read on.

Hand Washing: What Kind of Soap?

Although hand hygiene is considered so beneficial today, it is not always practiced. Hospital infections are some of the most common and serious medical complications: every year, almost 2 million patients in the United States acquire an infection when they are hospitalized, and 90,000 patients die from a hospital infection. Among the reasons for hospital infections is poor and inconsistent hand washing. In fact, according to the Centers for Disease Control and Prevention (CDC), appropriate hand washing is done only 40 percent of the time in hospitals.

The same is true outside the hospital. Studies in the United States have shown that hand washing is often not second nature for many people. Here are the results of studies indicating the proportion of women and men who wash their hands

- after using a public toilet: 90 percent of women, 75 percent of men
- before eating or cooking: 82 percent of women, 71 percent of men
- after changing a baby diaper: 82 percent of women, 64 percent of men
- after playing with a cat or dog: 50 percent of women, 34 percent of men
- after handling money: 27 percent of women, 14 percent of men

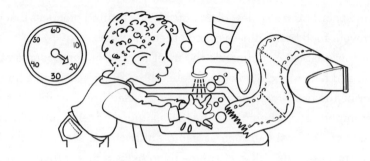

In addition, only one-third of adults wash their hands after coughing or sneezing into them. If adults are so poor at following such a basic hygiene rule, imagine how children fare. The CDC recommends hand hygiene as *the single most effective way* to prevent infections. Several products are available for hand hygiene: bar soap, liquid soap, alcohol-based hand gels and foams, and antibacterial soaps. Which should you use to wash your children's (and your own) hands?

Plain Soap

Plain soap removes germs mechanically with its detergent action. In effect, the ingredients in plain soap bind to dirt particles and organic material so that they can be rinsed off the hands with water. Many studies confirm the valuable preventive action of plain soap. For example, at U.S. day-care centers, introducing hand washing with water and plain soap decreased the incidence of diarrhea by 25 to 50 percent and of vomiting illnesses by 65 percent. At U.S. and Canadian schools, hand washing with water and plain soap decreased school absences due to infections in general by 25 percent. Absences specifically for respiratory infections decreased by 20 percent, and absences for gastrointestinal infections by 55 percent.

Results such as these have been reported from many other countries, too, including from developing countries with lower levels of hygiene. The World Health Organization estimates that, worldwide, good hand washing would save over 1 million children's lives each year, children who currently die from diarrhea and other infections. The WHO also declares that good hand washing with water and plain soap is "the most important measure to prevent infections."

I hope that by now you are convinced of the value of hand washing. Plain soap has wonderful results, but which is preferable, solid or liquid? Soap can itself become contaminated with germs, and because it has no antimicrobial ingredients, germs can survive on soap for a long time. In theory, then, soaps can spread germs. Studies have shown that solid soap in a soap dish is more likely to be contaminated than liquid soap. In U.S. hospitals and outpatient clinics, solid bar soap is no longer used.

Studies have not compared the frequency of infections in households that use solid versus liquid soap. If you use solid bar soap, however, place it on a grid container that does not retain water, instead of in a soap dish that holds potentially contaminated soapy water. If you use liquid soap, keep in mind that the container's plunger to express soap can also become contaminated. You should clean it with a sanitizing solution each time you clean taps and other bathroom fixtures, preferably every week.

Antibacterial Soap

Soaps that contain ingredients with antibacterial properties are widely available as both solid and liquid soaps; in fact, most liquid soaps in the U.S. market today are antibacterial. One can also buy laundry detergent, household cleaning products, deodorant, shampoo, lotion, and even cosmetics with antibacterial ingredients. These soaps and other products usually contain either triclosan or triclocarban, which are chemicals with antibacterial action that are considered antibiotics.

Many people wonder if antibacterial soaps are preferable to plain soaps. A recent study compared households using antibacterial soaps, detergents, and cleaning agents with households using plain, non-antibacterial products and found no difference in the frequency of infections in family members over the course of a year. This result is hardly surprising, given that most common infections are caused by viruses, not bacteria, and antibacterial soaps and cleaning products do not work against viruses. Moreover, as I discussed in chapter 8, the excessive use of antibiotics—an antibacterial soap is an antibiotic—may lead to selective growth of bacteria with antibiotic resistance.

In addition, triclosan and triclocarban are persistent environmental pollutants, meaning that they accumulate in the environment. Both have been detected in surface water. There are concerns that triclosan contains small quantities of toxic dioxins and can be converted into other dioxins in sunlight, and triclocarban is a suspected carcinogen. At the moment, the risk that these chemicals pose for human health is not clear. Because antibacterial soaps do not appear to lower the frequency of household infections and because they carry the theoretical risk of promoting antibiotic-resistant germs, the U.S. public health authorities recommend using plain soaps, plain detergents, and plain cleaning products at home, not ones with antibacterial action.

Hand-Sanitizing Gels

For various reasons, some people may avoid water and soap, or water and soap may not be available, but several alternate products are commercially available that neither require water nor dry the skin. Hand-sanitizing products such as foams and gels are very effective at killing microorganisms quickly. They also contain a moisturizing agent, so even with repeated use, they do not dry the skin.

Many of these products contain alcohol, although some contain chlorhexidine, iodine, or hexachlorophene. These ingredients kill many (but not all) microorganisms, including bacteria, fungi, and some viruses. A recent study from Finland and another from the United States examined the safety of alcohol-based sanitizing products for children. When these products were introduced in day-care centers as part of everyday hand cleaning for toddlers, the level of alcohol measured in both children and adults was very low, despite young children frequently putting their fingers in their mouths. These results are reassuring about the safety of alcohol-containing sanitizing products for children.

Hand-sanitizing products do not contain antimicrobials like triclosan or triclocarban, and they do not appear to contribute to antibiotic resistance. For this reason, and because they are often more acceptable than water and soap, they have been widely adopted for use in U.S. hospitals. The CDC recommends that health care workers use them in hospitals between patient contacts.

In laboratory studies, these products are much more effective than plain soap at removing bacteria and viruses from the skin, but there are

Effective Hand Washing, Step by Step

With soap and water:

1. Wet your hands and get some soap.
2. Rub your palms, the backs of your hands, and between the fingers and thumb for twenty seconds, or as long as it takes to sing "Twinkle, Twinkle, Little Star" or the ABCs.
3. Use water to rinse off the soap.
4. Dry your hands.

With a hand-sanitizing product:

1. Squirt the product onto your hands.
2. Rub your palms, the backs of your hands, and between the fingers and thumb until your hands are completely dry.

no clinical studies to prove that using these products lowers the frequency of infections compared with plain soap. These products are also effective for preventing influenza, including the new H1N1 influenza that became a pandemic in 2009. As a result of this pandemic, there has been a marked increase in the use of hand sanitizers.

Hand-sanitizing products are available commercially for household use, and I recommend that you carry one when you go out. If there is no sink available, then use the hand sanitizer to clean your children's hands before eating and when leaving school or the playground.

Beyond Hand Washing: Other Personal Hygiene Measures

Hand washing is critical, but it is by no means the only hygiene measure to instill in your children's repertoire. For example, it is better for children (and adults) to cough or sneeze into their elbow and not their hand, because germs are less likely to be spread to others from the elbow.

Touching other people, especially with kisses, is another way to transmit germs. All the germs found in the mouth—from rhinoviruses, which cause the common cold, to *Streptococcus*, which causes strep throat, to

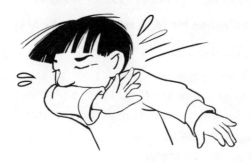

viruses and bacteria that cause meningitis—can be transmitted through kissing. From a microbial point of view, a kiss on the cheek or the scalp is safer for a child (and an adult) than a kiss on the lips. A hug is safer than a kiss. Perhaps the safest greeting is the Japanese practice of bowing instead of shaking hands.

Children should be taught not to share anything that comes into contact with their face or mouth, including toothpaste, toothbrushes, towels, tissues, and cups and glasses. For most people, having separate toothbrushes for each family member is obvious, but they may all share the same tube of toothpaste. Ideally, however, each person will have a separate tube of toothpaste. It is also a good idea for family members to have individual towels, because some germs, including the virus that causes hepatitis B, can be spread from a carrier to others by sharing towels. Other items that adolescents should not share with others are their razors, earrings, and makeup.

When it comes to dental hygiene, children often need a helping hand, and not just for the actual brushing. Toothbrushes should be rinsed with water after each use and should be placed upright to dry in the air, not in closed containers, and without touching other toothbrushes. Also, keep toothbrushes away from the toilet bowl, because a lot of germs vaporize into the surrounding air with every flush of the toilet. Get your child a new toothbrush every three to four months.

Antibacterial toothpaste and mouthwash have been shown to help prevent and treat gingivitis, which is a noncontagious inflammation of the gums caused by bacteria in the mouth. Recent studies suggest that gingivitis is one of the factors contributing to atherosclerosis (narrowing of the arteries) and heart disease as people age. No data support the notion that antibacterial toothpastes can prevent other infections spread through mouth secretions, such as colds, influenza, or strep throat. Antibacterial toothpastes are approved for use in children 6 years of age and older; there are no studies to verify their safety and effectiveness in younger children.

Many parents of toddlers despair that their child will never be toilet trained. But eventually children do learn to use the toilet, and they also need to learn how to clean themselves. Teach your children, especially daughters, to wipe themselves from the front to the back and never in the opposite direction. Careful wiping avoids transferring bacteria from the gut to the urethra, which can cause urinary tract infections.

If your adolescent daughter uses tampons, explain that she should change them frequently (four to five times a day) or alternate using tampons with using sanitary pads. She should avoid using super-absorbent tampons, because they can cause toxic shock syndrome, particularly when they have stayed in place for many hours. This syndrome is the result of bacteria accumulating and producing a toxin, and it can be life threatening. Young women who use tampons should be aware of the possible symptoms of toxic shock syndrome, which include nausea, weakness, dizziness, and rash. If they experience these symptoms, they should immediately remove the tampon and seek medical help.

Last, teach your children to avoid contact with other people's blood. If a friend or classmate grazes his knee, has a nosebleed, or loses a tooth, other children should ask the help of an adult instead of touching the blood-covered items themselves. The same is true if children find a needle or syringe in a park; teach them to never touch or play with these items. Some adolescents, or even younger children, may decide to exchange blood with a friend to become "blood brothers" or decide to give themselves a tattoo or piercing. None of these practices is safe; teach your children to avoid them.

Scrubbing and Scouring: Household Hygiene

Even though people believe, with good reason, that public places like schools, buses, public toilets, and restaurants are potential sources of microbes, their homes are not germ-free havens, either. The rooms in a house most likely to harbor germs are the kitchen, bathrooms, and the room of a person who is sick. In chapter 1, I wrote extensively about hygiene in the kitchen. For example, any surfaces that come into contact with raw meat and poultry should be cleansed with a sanitizing solution, such as a diluted bleach solution, and wiped with a paper towel. The source of one in five outbreaks of food poisoning is the home, most commonly the kitchen.

If one individual in a household is affected with *Salmonella*, then two of every three other household members will also acquire the germ, most likely from the toilet. Studies have shown that both the toilet seat and the toilet bowl carry *Salmonella* germs when a family member is infected with these bacteria. The same goes for rotavirus, the main viral cause of gastroenteritis in young children. This virus is excreted in huge numbers by an infected child (100 billion viruses per gram of feces), and it survives for days or even weeks on moist surfaces—not only in toilets, but on taps, sinks, and toys, too.

With all these potential germ hazards, what should you do to make your home safer? As with soaps and personal hygiene items, the great variety of household cleaners can be puzzling. There are plain detergents and cleaning products, as well as products that contain chemicals with sanitizing properties, such as chlorine bleach (which is a solution of 3 to 6 percent sodium hypochlorite), ammonia, alcohol, antibiotics, and phenols. Bleach is particularly effective at killing bacteria such as *Staphylococcus*, *Salmonella*, and *E. coli*. Note that bleach is not an antibiotic, so bacteria cannot develop resistance to it. Ammonia and phenols are less effective than bleach, but they do lower the number of bacteria. Plain detergents or those that contain baking soda, vinegar, and water do not kill germs; rather, they mechanically remove dirt.

When you are cleaning your home, pay particular attention to the following surfaces:

- Kitchen: sinks, taps, countertops, and possibly the floor
- Bathroom: toilet bowl and seat, sink, taps, bathtub, floor, and doorknob
- Baby's room: diaper-changing area and crib rail
- Sick child's room: all surfaces that the child or his secretions touch

Many people approach house cleaning by blitzing their whole house once a week or every fortnight. However, many experts recommend a more continual and targeted schedule of household cleaning:

- Kitchen sink and countertops: daily
- Bathroom sink, flush handles, and taps: once or twice a week
- Toilets, kitchen floor, and bathroom floor: weekly
- Sick child's room and bathroom: twice a day

This schedule is only a guide, of course. The key to living in a microbially safe home is to be aware of the areas of greatest microbial risk, which are the areas listed above, and to keep these areas clean all the time. In addition, pay attention to anything that comes into contact with hands or food, including dishrags, towels, cutting surfaces, kitchen appliances (including the fridge door handle), and mops. From a hygiene standpoint, cleaning floors is less important than cleaning other surfaces and fixtures, except if you have young children who crawl about on the floor and share the floor with pets. Of course, if the floor is contaminated with human secretions, then it needs to be cleaned.

When washing laundry, the machine cycles for delicate items use lower temperatures and less water than regular cycles, and they do not destroy bacteria that may be on clothes and linens. To lower the number of bacteria and viruses by 98 to 100 percent, use the hot water cycle and a laundry detergent containing bleach, and then completely dry the items, preferably in a dryer.

The practice of focused hygiene, as I describe here, maximizes your protection from pathogenic bacteria and viruses, while allowing a certain degree of exposure to nonpathogenic bacteria in the environment. In other words, it is impossible to live in a sterile home, so focus your efforts on getting rid of the most harmful microorganisms. You may wonder, however, if data show that adhering to strict rules of household hygiene or using sanitizing solutions actually decreases the incidence of infections. The answer is that very few studies have addressed this issue.

One recent study of 240 households (with an average of two to three children) in U.S. cities examined the effect of different ways and means of household cleaning on the frequency of the most common symptoms of infection, such as diarrhea, vomiting, fever, sore throat, sniffles, pink eye, and skin infections. The study found fewer symptoms of infections in households where a bleach detergent was used for the laundry and the hot water cycle for white clothes. It also found that people who drank bottled water in their home had more symptoms of infection than people who drank tap water. The reasons for this result are unclear; the researchers postulated that more than one family member may have drunk from the same bottle kept in the refrigerator.

The study also found that people who believed that germs are most likely to be found in the kitchen had half the frequency of infection symptoms compared with people who believed that germs are most likely to come from other places, such as toys, other people, toilets, or soiled clothes. This study did not, however, find a difference between households that used different types of cleaning products. The incidence of infection symptoms among people living in houses where sanitizing solutions, such as bleach, were used for cleaning did not differ from that among people in households using plain detergents.

Tap or Bottled? The Water We Drink

In the United States, the Environmental Protection Agency (EPA) regulates water quality in public water systems. In most homes, tap water comes from a public water system. Some homes are supplied by private wells, however, which are not regulated. In these cases, well owners are responsible for ensuring that the water is safe for drinking. Information about treating and testing well water is available on the EPA website (http://water.epa.gov/drink/).

Public water systems treat water with a series of purifying processes that include filtering and adding sanitizing substances, such as chlorine. There has been great progress in drinking water treatment, and outbreaks from contaminated municipal water are infrequent, but the risks have not been eliminated completely. For example, in 1993, there was a large outbreak of infection with the parasite *Cryptosporidium*, which contaminated municipal water in Wisconsin and resulted in illness for four hundred thousand individuals and forty deaths among people with a weakened immune system. As I discussed in chapter 3, chlorination of water does not destroy *Cryptosporidium*; this parasite can only be removed by special filters. After the 1993 outbreak, the U.S. public health authorities developed new regulations for the safety of tap water, and the regulations came into effect in 2006.

Several consumer groups have expressed concerns about the safety of some water treatment methods, especially the use of chlorine as a sanitizer. Chlorine is a very effective water sanitizer, but it does react chemically with the water, resulting in the formation of byproducts. The long-term safety of these chemical byproducts is not known. Some critics claim that consuming them over prolonged periods might lead to a higher risk of cancer or other conditions. The tap water treatment regulations currently in effect do include measures to limit people's exposure to such byproducts.

Every year, U.S. citizens consume more and more bottled water. Some of the products on the market (about a quarter of bottled waters) are tap water that has undergone further processing, so the water has in fact been subjected to tap water sanitation procedures. The rest of the bottled water products come from underground springs. Spring water is thought to be less likely to be contaminated with germs and so may not undergo the same sanitation procedures as surface water. The Food and Drug Administration regulates bottled water as a packaged food, but the rules for testing microbial contamination levels are more lax for bottled waters than for EPA-regulated tap water. In general, tap water undergoes stricter procedures of testing and sanitation, which makes it generally safer from a microbial standpoint. Still, spread of infections from bottled water is a rare event in the United States.

Some people use commercially available filters to further clean tap water. Some refrigerator-freezers incorporate filters, too. None of these filters has been proven to decrease the incidence of infections at home. Tap water from public water systems has already been filtered, and most germs have been removed. Further filtering or purifying might remove some toxins and chemicals, but to date, studies have produced nonconclusive results. Hospitals use water filters to remove the bacterium *Legionella*, which can lead to a dangerous form of pneumonia in older or immunosuppressed individuals; this bacterium is not usually a concern for healthy people in their homes.

If everyone in your family is healthy, and nobody has a weakened immune system, further purification of tap water is unnecessary. If a member of your household does have a weakened immune system, your doctor can advise you about the safest choice.

Fresh Air? The Air We Breathe

Parents are often very concerned about the quality of air their children breathe, particularly in large cities and industrial areas. In terms of microorganisms, the air is not really dangerous. Generally speaking, aerating your house with outdoor air is a healthy habit that lowers the risk of infections that can be spread indoors.

However, there are a few instances when air quality can be compromised by microorganisms. If the air is filled with large amounts of dust, such as from nearby excavations or construction zones or from dust storms, there is a risk of fungal spores becoming airborne. Some fungal spores can cause pneumonia, but these infections are mostly limited to people with weakened immune systems. In addition, indoor air can be contaminated by mold spores, typically in areas of high humidity, such as in a flooded basement, in areas with leaking water pipes, or in showers with excessive steam. Inhaled mold spores can cause allergies, including asthma, sneezing, irritation of the eyes, and other symptoms, or, rarely, pneumonia (mostly in people with weakened immune responses).

Filters and other devices to clean indoor air can lower the levels of molds and help to decrease asthma symptoms caused by allergenic substances in mold. In hospitals, high-efficiency particulate air (HEPA) filters are used to remove microscopic particles from the air in intensive care, oncology, and transplantation units, where even a small number of germs can be hazardous for the very vulnerable patients. HEPA filters have become available for home use too, but to date, no data suggest that their use decreases the incidence of infections at home, school, or other places where healthy individuals spend their time.

For years pediatricians have been recommending that parents use vaporizers and cool mist humidifiers to relieve the symptoms of common colds, croup, pneumonia, and sinusitis. However, studies have failed to prove that such devices are effective in relieving these symptoms.

If you do use one of these devices, be sure to clean it frequently. Vaporizers and humidifiers can themselves become colonized with potentially harmful bacteria, like *Pseudomonas* and other germs that grow in moist conditions.

A 2007 study showed that dry air promotes the spread of influenza. However, studies have not yet addressed the question of whether it would be beneficial to humidify indoor air in places like emergency rooms and nursing homes, where the spread of influenza might be linked to a higher risk of complications.

Another recent study found that environmental pollutants in the air, such as carbon monoxide, nitrous oxide, sulfur dioxide, and particulate matter, are significantly correlated with ear infections in children. I cannot mention environmental pollutants and air quality without discussing smoking. The health risks of passive smoking have been repeatedly shown in many studies. Apart from the increased risks of lung cancer, allergies, asthma, and sudden infant death, inhaling second-hand smoke has infectious risks. Children exposed to cigarette smoke have an increased incidence of ear infections and respiratory infections, including bronchitis, bronchiolitis, and pneumonia. Even a fetus exposed to maternal smoking in the womb is more likely to contract these infections during early childhood.

The Hygiene Hypothesis

In the 1980s, scientists observed that eczema and allergic rhinitis (hay fever) were less common in children who came from large families. In 1989, an English researcher, David Strachan, proposed the hygiene hypothesis to explain this observation. Strachan reasoned that children from large families probably had greater exposure to germs through their many siblings, compared with children from families with only one child and consequently a "cleaner" environment. Later, other researchers suggested an increase in autoimmune disorders could also be explained by the hygiene hypothesis. This hypothesis has sparked a lot of interest among epidemiologists and immunologists, as well as among the general public, judging from the number of newspaper and magazine articles and books, frequently with sensational titles, that have been published on the subject. The scientific evidence that forms the basis of the theory, however, is still controversial.

It is undisputed that allergic conditions, such as asthma and hay fever, are on the rise. Epidemiological data show that in the last thirty years or so, the incidence of asthma has more than doubled. Autoimmune disorders, in which the body attacks itself—for example, lupus, ulcerative colitis, Crohn's disease, and several others—are also increasing. The reason for the greater frequency of these conditions used to be attributed to environmental pollution or toxins in food. However, scientists also observed that allergies were more common in people who lived in microbiologically cleaner environments. Developed countries have a higher incidence of allergic and autoimmune disorders than developing countries. Studies have shown that as countries with limited resources become more prosperous, and consequently, microbially "cleaner," there is an increase in the number of immune disorder diagnoses.

In the 1990s, before the unification of Germany, the incidence of allergies was much higher in West Germany, which enjoyed a higher per capita income and overall higher living standards compared with East Germany. In Africa and Asia, where the hygiene level is lower than in Europe and North America, the incidence of allergic and autoimmune disorders is very low.

Could genetic factors be responsible? It is possible, but there is some evidence against this suggestion. For example, when Southeast Asians immigrate to Western countries, the incidence of allergic and autoimmune disorders increases to Western levels within one generation. Clearly, genetic factors alone cannot explain this phenomenon.

The hygiene hypothesis proposes that our immune system needs exposure to a number of germs and a certain level of dirt in the environment in order to develop normally. By cleaning the environment excessively and preventing many infections, our immune system may not encounter the necessary stimuli to learn what really constitutes an enemy. According to the hypothesis, such a misguided immune system may react against harmless environmental antigens to cause allergies or against the body to cause autoimmune disorders.

A more detailed description of the hygiene hypothesis involves the way in which the immune system responds to the ocean of harmless bacteria in our environment, and how it learns to tolerate these bacteria with the help of a type of white blood cell called *regulatory T lymphocytes*. Regulatory T lymphocytes have the job of regulating certain immune system responses so that the immune system stays balanced. According to the hypothesis, if a person does not encounter a "normal" level of bacteria in the environment, his body does not produce the necessary levels of immune regulatory factors, resulting in overreaction to many stimuli.

Supporters of the hygiene hypothesis suggest that antibiotics may contribute to an overly clean environment. Other supporters claim that vaccines keep children "too clean" and suggest that children should be exposed to the infections rather than be vaccinated.

To date, there is little evidence that the hygiene hypothesis is scientifically valid. Some biological experiments support the hygiene hypothesis, but so far they are few and weak. For example, in one study, mice susceptible to type 1 diabetes (an autoimmune disorder) were less likely to develop the condition if they had been experimentally infected with a particular parasite. In another study, a small number of patients with serious inflammatory colitis were infected with helminth parasites (a type of worm), which are harmless for humans, and this therapeutic infection improved their colitis symptoms. In addition, one study reported a correlation between the use of antibiotics during a baby's first year and an increased chance of asthma; however, the correlation was weak, and even the study's authors noted that the results should be interpreted with caution. One factor, though, that has been found repeatedly to correlate with a lower incidence of allergies is exposure at a young age to an environment containing farm animals such as sheep and cattle.

Although the hygiene hypothesis might have biological plausibility, many other factors could play a role beyond differences in hygiene level. For example, perhaps in the West we have the knowledge and means to diagnose allergic and autoimmune disorders better than in poorer countries. Also, some people have wondered if it is truly possible to have sterilized the environment to such a degree that children's immune systems cannot learn which substances are enemies and which are not. In fact, more children are attending out-of-home child care from a very early age and therefore are exposed to more germs than they were a generation ago. Indeed, studies in children attending day-care centers that followed an enhanced hygiene schedule and frequent hand washing did not show a rise in allergies or asthma compared with children in day-care centers that had more lax hygiene standards.

Currently, many scientists believe that our immune system "learns" at a young age to tolerate many harmless environmental germs, such as mycobacteria and lactobacilli, that are found in large quantities (or were in the past) in water and food, as well as helminth parasites. The continuous existence of these types of microbes in the environment is thought to lead to the activation of immunoregulatory cells that repress immune responses, including responses against antigens both in the body itself and in the environment. The absence of such germs from the environment may lead to a lowering of immune regulation, with a subsequent increase in immune reactions and overreactions.

Should you then follow the advice of some of the articles and books proclaiming that it is good for children to "eat dirt"? Keep in mind that so far, the hygiene hypothesis is just that—a hypothesis. I recommend that you teach your children to wash their hands before eating and after using the toilet, keep your environment clean, vaccinate your children with the recommended vaccines, and give them antibiotics when necessary (and only when necessary). These practices will keep both your children and you healthy.

Thanks to progress in medicine and public health, we do not live in an era of cholera epidemics from drinking water, crippling polio from a lack of vaccines, and other dreadful infectious diseases. Nobody wants to return to such an era. We know that infections and the resultant inflammation do not benefit our long-term health. Rather, inflammation contributes to conditions such as atherosclerosis, coronary artery disease, arthritis, and cancer, and it shortens survival. We also know that a proven practice for reducing the chance of childhood asthma is to stop smoking, especially around children.

Several large studies currently under way are trying to get some more answers. The European Union is sponsoring a study in European countries with different levels of living and hygiene standards and with only small genetic differences, such as Finland, Estonia, and Russia. This study will follow thousands of children for several years and will record data on hygiene parameters, diet, infections, and the bacterial content of the children's intestines to examine correlations with the development of allergic disorders. In the United States, a similar study, recently started, will follow one hundred thousand children for twenty-one years to explore many questions related to the causes of allergies and environmental diseases. It will certainly be interesting to see how the hygiene hypothesis plays out over the next several years.

─────────────────── ┤ MAIN POINTS ├ ───────────────────
Measures to Avoid Infections with Good Hygiene

- Teach your children good personal hygiene habits, including not sharing personal items, coughing and sneezing into the elbow, and washing hands frequently.
- Teach your children to wash their hands
  - before eating,
  - after using the toilet,
  - after coughing or sneezing in their hand and after wiping their nose,
  - after returning home from school, playing with other children, parties, sports activities, or shopping,
  - after playing with pets, and
  - after playing with a sick child or touching a sick child's toys.
- Wash hands (yours and your children's) with warm water and plain soap for fifteen to twenty seconds, or as long as it takes to sing "Twinkle, Twinkle, Little Star." There is no need to use antibacterial soap.
- When you are not near a sink, use an alcohol-based hand sanitizer.
- When the hands are visibly soiled, use water and soap, if possible, rather than a hand sanitizer.
- Be aware of the areas in the home that carry the greatest microbial risks (primarily the kitchen, bathroom, and sick person's room) and keep these areas clean at all times.

Myths and Truths

DOES SCIENCE BACK UP TRADITIONAL WISDOM ABOUT PREVENTING INFECTIONS?

As children, many of us repeatedly heard advice about how to prevent and treat colds and other infections, advice that, as parents, we often repeat to our own children. New parents are often bombarded with suggestions from well-meaning but interfering grandmothers, mothers, neighbors, or friends. Even though we may doubt the validity of some past practices, many of them have survived numerous generations and are found in cultures around the world. So perhaps they truly are of some benefit. In this chapter, I discuss some of the more widespread and oft-repeated folk beliefs and practices about preventing and treating childhood infections, primarily the common cold, but also some others.

Coats, Scarves, and Umbrellas: Cold Weather and the Common Cold

The belief that colds are caused by cold temperatures is widespread and found in many different nations. Even the words we use—common cold—to name the (mostly viral) infections of the upper respiratory system indicate this belief, and this linguistic link occurs in many languages.

The belief that the cold causes colds likely stems from two factors: first, the belief originated at a time before germs were recognized as the cause of infectious diseases, a discovery made in the first decades of the twentieth century. Indeed, the 1950s and 1960s were the golden age for virology, with scientists discovering hundreds of viruses and developing vaccines against several of them, such as polio and measles. It was not until 1956 that the first rhinoviruses (the most common causes of common colds) were discovered and grown in the laboratory.

Second, respiratory tract infections are undeniably much more frequent during the cold fall and winter months of the year. Many viruses have seasonal cycles and spread more when outdoor temperatures are lower. In contrast to many other viruses, rhinoviruses replicate better in lower temperatures; these viruses frequently replicate in the nose, which has a lower temperature than the body's core. The influenza virus, which also targets the respiratory tract, is transmitted through small droplets and spreads more t lower outside temperature, and lower humidity, as well. During warmer months, influenza spreads only through direct contact with contaminated objects or very close contact with a sick individual. Neither route is as efficient as transmission through small droplets, which can span a distance of up to three feet. Thus, influenza epidemics in temperate climates usually occur in the fall and winter and rarely in the summer. Higher crowding indoors and in schools also promotes the spread of upper respiratory infections during winter months.

You may wonder whether your children will be less susceptible to colds if you dress them warmly and keep them dry or if you wrap a scarf around their nose when it is cold outside. Such a study has not been performed. Indeed, only a few studies have examined whether cold temperatures cause respiratory infections.

In one small study done more than forty years ago, in 1968, researchers experimentally infected forty-nine volunteers' noses with a rhinovirus. Then one-third of the volunteers were exposed to cold temperatures, either in a cold room (40°F) or a cold bath (90°F), at various times after infection: while incubating the illness, while experiencing clinical symptoms, or while convalescing. Volunteers in all groups, both those exposed to cold temperature and those not exposed, developed symptoms of a common cold. The symptoms lasted for the same duration and were equally serious, and all volunteers developed antibodies in their blood (a marker of immunity).

More recently, in 2005, researchers at the Center for the Common Cold at the University of Cardiff, Wales, studied 180 volunteers who did not have symptoms of a common cold. Ninety of the volunteers placed

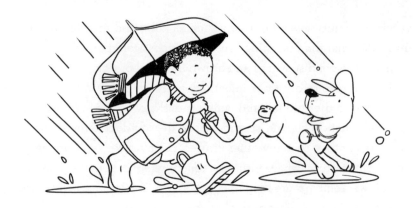

their bare feet in a bucket of ice water for twenty minutes, while ninety placed their feet, wearing socks and shoes, in an empty bucket. None of the volunteers had cold symptoms before or immediately after the experiment, yet twenty-six of the ninety volunteers who had placed their feet in ice water (29 percent, or almost one-third) developed symptoms of a common cold in the subsequent five days, compared with only eight of ninety (9 percent) who were not exposed to cold water.

How is it possible that exposing the feet to ice water for twenty minutes can cause an upper respiratory infection? The researchers hypothesized that the volunteers developed common cold symptoms because their immune defenses may have been lowered by exposure to cold temperature or because the many viruses that we all encounter and that often remain subclinical (do not cause overt symptoms) may have replicated more easily thanks to lower body temperature. Proving these hypotheses would be difficult. The study did not examine which viruses caused the volunteers to become ill, and it relied on subjective responses to a questionnaire asking the volunteers to describe their symptoms. (A more objective measure would quantify, or count, a related parameter, such as the number of tissues a person used.) Thus, it is possible that the volunteers who had been exposed to a cold temperature remembered, emphasized, or mentioned more frequently their symptoms because of conscious or subconscious associations made between cold temperatures and common cold symptoms.

Last, some studies have experimentally exposed animals to extreme cold (much colder than in the studies described above with human volunteers) and have repeatedly shown a correlation between exposure to extreme cold, as well as other forms of biological stress, and increased frequency and severity of infections.

Overall, the available data to causally associate cold temperatures with the common cold are few and weak. But data to reject a link between the two do not exist either. Therefore, I recommend that you dress your children warmly when it is cold outside, and you keep them dry when it is raining. Perhaps more important, though, remind them to wash their hands and to avoid close contact with people who have symptoms of an upper respiratory infection.

The Importance of Getting Enough Sleep

We have all heard or read that sleep is critical for proper development in children, for maintaining good health, and even for preventing and treating infections. Does science support this belief, and if your children do not get enough sleep, will they be more vulnerable to infections?

Sleep and sleep deprivation affect numerous immune and endocrine (hormone) circuits in the body. Many laboratory studies have shown that sleep affects various types of cells in the immune system, as well as the production of antibodies and cytokines (proteins that act as messengers in the immune system). These cells and processes are also affected by sleep deprivation. Some of the molecules produced by the immune system can, in turn, affect sleep-wake cycles. For example, someone who is sick or has a fever tends to sleep more, which is the result of cytokines that directly regulate sleep. While a sick person sleeps, her immune system secretes higher levels of other cytokines that fight the pathogenic organisms. Thus, there is a scientific basis to the belief that it is beneficial to get enough sleep when the body is fighting a cold or other infection.

In studies performed with laboratory animals, sleep deprivation (and other forms of biological stress, such as very intense physical exercise) led to more serious or even life-threatening infections when these animals were infected experimentally. It is difficult to extrapolate from the results of such studies in laboratory animals to humans, because many environmental factors (diet, exercise, exposure to pathogenic germs, state of health) differ from person to person and are difficult to control. Other factors, including crowding and stress, are also at play.

Findings from recent clinical studies indicate that even a small decrease in the length of time that people sleep can increase susceptibility to infections. Young, healthy volunteers participated in a study where one group slept for only four hours every night for a week, while a second group slept for the more usual eight hours per night. After the fourth night, both groups received the influenza vaccine. Ten days later, the researchers measured antibodies that had developed in the blood as a result of vaccination. The volunteers who slept for four hours per night had half the amount of antibodies against influenza compared with the volunteers who slept eight hours per night. One month after receiving the vaccine, however, volunteers in both groups had the same amounts of antibodies.

These preliminary and limited results indicate that lack of sleep can indeed affect the body's susceptibility to infections and, to a certain extent, the body's ability to respond to infections. For many more reasons related to their health and cognitive development, your children need to sleep at least eight to twelve hours every night, with the number of hours depending on their age.

Chicken Soup: Food for Health?

Many mothers and grandmothers swear by chicken soup as the ultimate food for a child who is sick, from the common cold and influenza to a range of other illnesses. People around the world share this opinion, and it even surfaces from centuries ago. In the twelfth century, the physician and philosopher Maimonides wrote in his book *On the Causes of Symptoms* that the meat of a hen or rooster and their broth are beneficial for restoring health.

Perhaps not surprisingly, clinical studies have not examined the benefits of soup for preventing or treating infections in people. Is there any biological basis to the belief? Colds are caused by many different viruses, so if soup does have an effect, it should be on a mechanism common to all these viruses. Possible mechanisms include soup providing liquid to the body, and its warm vapors helping to unblock nasal passages.

In addition to prescribing chicken soup, many people give hot beverages, such as warmed milk, hot tea, chamomile, or cocoa to people with a cold or sore throat. Their therapeutic benefits have no scientific basis, but, as for chicken soup, they offer soothing warmth, and they do not cause any harm.

Rubs, Inhalations, and Other Folk Remedies

Inhaling various herbs or rubbing herbal concoctions on the skin are also ancient remedies for the common cold, sinusitis, and asthma. Herbs such as eucalyptus oil, camphor, menthol, oregano, rosemary, and sage continue to be used among many countries of the Mediterranean region and Central and South America. Studies in the United States have shown that folk remedies are commonly used here, too, although their use differs by ethnic group.

The use of herbs may have a scientific basis, because some of them have antibacterial and antiviral action as well as an effect on the cough reflex and blood flow to the nasal cavities. In fact, laboratory animals that inhaled various herbs showed improved lung function. No clinical studies, however, examined their benefit for people with a common cold.

Camphor is an aromatic, volatile substance that has been used for hundreds of years in the folk remedies of many cultures to treat the common cold and other conditions, and it is still used in lotions, oils, and inhalations. Camphor is one ingredient in Vicks Vaporub (at a concentration of 4.8 percent; other ingredients are 2.6 percent menthol and 1.2 percent eucalyptus oil). Camphor causes a local sensation of heat and mild numbness, and many people connect its characteristic potent smell with "strong medicine." A recent study suggested a greater improvement in congestion, cough, and sleep in children with upper respiratory infections who used Vicks Vaporub compared with a placebo product.

You need to be careful with camphor-containing products, however, because camphor can be toxic for the liver. Absorbing it through the skin has led to liver toxicity and seizures, particularly in babies and young children. To be available on the market in the United States, preparations that contain camphor must have a concentration of less than 11 percent. In other countries, however, a similar restriction may not be in place. Vicks preparations are safe to apply on the skin, but children have been poisoned by accidentally ingesting a large quantity. I recommend that you do not use camphor products for the common cold in children younger than 2 years, because these products' effectiveness is unproved, and they can have toxic side effects.

In general, most folk remedies for the common cold and other common minor ailments are harmless, and some even have limited scientific support of an effect. They can certainly supplement medical practice and your doctor's advice. If you want to use any supplemental therapies for your children, discuss them with your doctor, because some herbs or other remedies may have interactions with medications that your children might need to take. Your doctor can give you guidance on which remedies are appropriate and which to avoid.

⊢ MAIN POINTS ⊢
Measures to Safely Use Folk Remedies

- Be aware that although most folk remedies and beliefs about treating common colds and other minor childhood ailments are harmless, there are some exceptions, notably the use of camphor.
- Speak to your doctor before giving your children herbs or other remedies, in case of possible interactions with medical treatments. Herbal remedies may have no or only a small effect, but sometimes they can supplement medical treatment.

Afterword

In this book, I have given you information and facts from up-to-date science in the fields of pediatrics and infectious diseases so that you have the knowledge to understand and prevent infections in your children, and indeed in your whole family. In the current era of rapid changes in sociopolitics, human population, climate, and ecology, the balance between humans and the microbial world has been disrupted. During the last three decades, many new infections have appeared, such as HIV infection, variant Creutzfeldt-Jakob disease (the human equivalent of bovine spongiform encephalopathy, or mad cow disease), severe acute respiratory syndrome (SARS), and avian and swine influenzas, to mention only a few.

From the 1970s to today, scientists have identified over thirty new pathogenic microorganisms. Scientific and medical research have also discovered infectious agents to be the cause of many conditions with previously elusive origins, resulting in a true revolution for treatment. For example, when I was in medical school, stomach ulcers were considered a chronic noninfectious disease, attributed to a combination of stress, poor dietary habits, overproduction of stomach acid, and genetic factors. Now we know that in the majority of cases, a bacterium, *Helicobacter pylori*, causes stomach ulcers. Treatment has evolved from milk and crackers to antibiotics, which prevent stomach cancer as well as treating the ulcers. Current data suggest that, in the future, diseases such as atherosclerotic heart disease, some neurological and psychiatric conditions, diabetes, and others may also prove to be caused by microbes.

It is clear today that we are far from declaring victory over or closing the chapter on infections, as some scientists had announced some years

233

ago—erroneously, it turns out. Even with today's extraordinary technologies, infectious diseases cause more deaths worldwide than any other type of disease. The great scientific advances of the twentieth century, mainly the discovery of antibiotics and vaccines, as well as the tremendous progress in hygiene and public health, gave many people a false sense of security and the arrogance to think that humans are more clever than microorganisms. Yet, it did not take long for microbes to develop mechanisms to resist most of our antibiotics. Having existed on Earth for over 3 billion years, vastly longer than humans, it is not surprising that microbes continue to challenge us. Diseases that we considered under control, such as tuberculosis and malaria, are making a comeback, because the germs that cause them have developed resistance to antibiotics. Diseases such as poliomyelitis, that had been almost eliminated from the world, are resurging, because we have not used the available vaccines as much as we could have.

Social and demographic changes, such as urbanization, crowding, and widespread use of day care have increased exposure to infections, in particular infections transmitted through the air. Increases in air travel and immigration also bring us in contact with infections from other countries. Climate change, with warming temperatures and increasing frequency of extreme weather phenomena, might in the future bring to the United States infections that today are considered tropical. In addition, today's sexual mores are evolving in a way that promotes the spread of sexually transmitted diseases. Longer life expectancy, aging, and the increased survival of patients with cancer and on immunosuppressive therapies, as well as new immunosuppressive diseases such as AIDS, have made the population as a whole more susceptible to many infectious diseases.

A change in our thinking is then in order. We should consider ourselves—human beings—not as isolated organisms but as ecosystems of multiple organisms. Microorganisms are part of the ecosystem and always will be. In effect, we "swim" in a sea of microbes, most of which coexist symbiotically with humans, that is, with mutual benefit, through mechanisms that have evolved over a long time. There is no sense in declaring war on microbes. Humans are unlikely to be victorious, and worse, such a war would cause irreparable damage to the ecosystem balance and to the multiple benefits for human health achieved over millennia of coexistence.

On the other hand, by taking advantage of the benefits of "good" germs, the infectious diseases medicine of the future can focus on fighting only the pathogenic bacteria while preserving the harmless and beneficial ones. Only by restoring the balance between humans and microorganisms will science and medicine be able to find solutions for infections and to correct the modern epidemics of allergy and autoimmunity. In the future, these conditions and disorders may prove to be a result of the massive destruction of harmless microorganisms by "bombs," such as wide-spectrum antibiotics, when what we need are "bullets" to target specific germs.

In today's world, we receive massive amounts of information from television, newspapers, magazines, and the Internet. As parents, we try to filter and decipher the barrage of information to keep our children safe and healthy. It can often be difficult to know which sources to trust when you hear or read about a new disease or magic bullet. One study of medical information that was found through commonly used Internet search engines reported that only 40 percent of hits for a particular query provided reliable information. Many websites are unreliable or out-of-date, while others aim at commercial profit. In addition, the numerous blogs and chat rooms on the Internet often offer personal views and anecdotes rather than scientifically proven data. Freely accessed encyclopedias are not necessarily accurate either. Clearly, we all need to be prudent and critically evaluate the information we receive, whether it is from the Internet or other media sources.

Medical and scientific research proceeds in a series of small steps, so it takes time for experiments to be repeated and reproduced by others in order to establish which discoveries and facts prove reliable. The nature of news journalism, on the other hand, means that reporters do not have the luxury of waiting so long. Instead of paying attention to dramatic news headlines, wait to see whether a new finding is confirmed by ongoing scientific research and listen to scientists' commentaries.

Good sources of information about medical issues are your physician and reliable websites such as those produced by many medical and public health organizations. The American Academy of Pediatrics (AAP), the

National Institutes of Health (NIH), and the Centers for Disease Control and Prevention (CDC) as well as most major medical centers and medical schools offer various online resources and information about infectious diseases and practical advice on prevention and treatment. (See also the listing of trustworthy Web resources at the end of this book.) In addition, in the bibliography, I have included the titles of other books that can further guide you and answer many of your questions.

I hope that you will embrace the main messages that I convey in this book. It is impossible for our children to avoid germs altogether. The body's immune system is constantly making contact with the microbial world, and in most cases, the interaction is beneficial, keeping the good germs in their places and maintaining the immune system in a state of calm vigilance. The keys to minimizing the impact of bad germs on your children's health are to be consistent with good hygiene practices, to use antibiotics properly and judiciously, and to make use of vaccines. With these basic practices and the other information throughout the book, you will know what to apply in your daily routines and what to teach to your children. Thus, you can lower the number of infections that your children contract and maximize their health.

I do not believe in oversimplification, but I distill the message of this book as:

- *No* to overprotecting your children from germs
- *No* to the use of antimicrobial soaps and cleaning products at home
- *No* to the excessive use of antibiotics
- *Yes* to strategic hand washing with water and soap (or with an alcohol-based gel when water is not easily accessible)
- *Yes* to being conscious of germs and the pathways they use to travel and replicate both inside and outside the home
- *Yes* to vaccines

The fact that you have read this book means that you would like to learn as much as possible and do what is best for your family. You are certainly on the right path. Finding the correct information, evaluating it critically, understanding our dynamic balance with germs, and applying focused prevention practices will help you and your children successfully swim the microbial sea.

Trustworthy Web Resources

American Academy of Pediatrics
www.aap.org

American College of Sports Medicine
www.acsm.org

Association of Professional Piercers
www.safepiercing.org

Centers for Disease Control and Prevention
www.cdc.gov/foodnet
www.cdc.gov/foodsafety

Environmental Working Group
www.foodnews.org/walletguide.php

Food Safety and Inspection Service, U.S. Department of Agriculture
www.fsis.usda.gov

Infectious Diseases Society of America
www.idsociety.org

Johns Hopkins University's Institute for the Safety of Vaccines
www.vaccinesafety.edu

National Institutes of Health
www.nih.gov

National Library of Medicine's Medline Plus
www.medlineplus.gov

Partnership for Food Safety Education
www.fightbac.org

U.S. Environmental Protection Agency (ground water and drinking water)
http://water.epa.gov/drink/

World Health Organization (travel and vaccine information)
www.who.int

Selected Bibliography

General

American Academy of Pediatrics. Immunizations and infectious diseases. Fischer MC, Editor in Chief, American Academy of Pediatrics, Elk Grove Village, IL, 2006.

Institute of Medicine. Emerging infections. Microbial threats to health in the United States. Lederberg J, Shope RE, Oaks SC, Editors. National Academy Press, Washington, DC, 1992.

Offit PA, Bell LM. Vaccines: What you should know. 3rd Edition. John Wiley & Sons, Hoboken, NJ, 2003.

Principle and practice of pediatric infectious diseases. Long SS, Pickering LK, Prober CG, Editors. Churchill Livingstone Elsevier, Third Edition, 2008.

Red Book. 2006 report of the Committee on Infectious Diseases. 27th Edition. American Academy of Pediatrics, Elk Grove Village, IL, 2006.

Rotbart HA, MD. Germ proof your kids. The complete guide to protecting (without overprotecting) your family from infections. ASM Press, Washington, DC, 2008.

Ryder CS. Take your pediatrician with you. Keeping your child healthy at home and on the road. Johns Hopkins University Press, Baltimore, MD, 2007.

Sherman IW. Twelve diseases that changed our world. ASM Press, Washington, DC, 2007.

Snyder Sachs J. Good germs, bad germs. Health and survival in a bacterial world. Hill and Wang, New York, 2007.

Chapter 1. I'm Hungry! Food-Borne Germs and Food Preparation Safety

American Academy of Pediatrics. Guide to your child's nutrition. Making peace at the table and building healthy eating habits for life. Dietz WH, Stern L, Editors. Villard, New York, 1999.

Collignon P. Resistant Escherichia coli—We are what we eat. Clinical Infectious Diseases 2009;49:202-3.

Denno DM, Keene WE, Hutter CM, et al. Tri-county comprehensive assessment of risk factors for sporadic reportable bacterial enteric infection in children. Journal of Infectious Diseases 2009;199:467–76.

Entis P. Food safety. Old habits, new perspectives. American Society for Microbiology Press, Washington, DC, 2007.

Chapter 2. A, B, C and 1, 2, 3: Common Germs at Day Care and School

Managing infectious diseases in child care and schools. A quick reference guide. 2nd Edition. Aronson SS and Shope TR, Editors, American Academy of Pediatrics, Elk Grove Village, IL, 2009.

Shaman J, Kohn M. Absolute humidity modulates influenza survival, transmission, and seasonality. PNAS Early Edition February 2009:1–6.

Chapter 3. Swim, Ski, or Wrestle: Germs Encountered When Playing Sports

Infections of leisure. Schlossberg D, Editor. 3rd Edition, ASM Press, Washington, DC, 2004.

Kirkland EB, Adams BB. Methicillin-resistant Staphylococcus aureus and athletes. J Am Acad Dermatol 2008;59:494–502.

Chapter 5. The Great Outdoors: Germs in the Garden, at the Campground, on the Farm, and at the Beach

Holve S. Envenomations. In: Nelson textbook of pediatrics, Behrman RE, Kliegman RM, Jenson HB, Editors. 16th Edition. Saunders, Philadelphia, 2000.

Infections of leisure. Schlossberg D, Editor. 3rd Edition, ASM Press, Washington, DC, 2004.

Ryder CS. Take your pediatrician with you. Keeping your child healthy at home and on the road. Johns Hopkins University Press, Baltimore, MD, 2007.

Tahmassebi JF, O'Sullivan EA. A case report of an unusual mandibular swelling in a 4-year-old child possibly caused by a jellyfish sting. International Journal of Paediatric Dentistry 1998;8:51–54.

Chapter 6. Close to Home and Overseas: Tips for Avoiding Germs When You Travel

Centers for Disease Control and Prevention. Travelers' health—yellow book. Arguin PM, Kozarsky PE, Reed C, Editors. Elsevier, Philadelphia, 2007.

World Health Organization. International travel and health. 2008.

Chapter 8. Taking Medicine: The Use and Misuse of Antibiotics

ESAC. Scientific evaluation on the use of antimicrobial agents in human therapy. www.esac.ua.ac.be, accessed April 1, 2009.

Goossens H, Ferech M, Vander Stichele R, Elseviers M, for the ESAC Project Group.

Outpatient antibiotic use in Europe and association with resistance: A cross-national database study. Lancet 2005;365:579–86.

van de Sande-Bruinsma N, Grundmann H, Verloo D, et al. Antimicrobial drug use and resistance in Europe. Emerging Infectious Diseases 2008;14:1722–30.

Chapter 9. The Miracle of Modern Prevention:
Vaccine Safety and Effectiveness

American Academy of Pediatrics. Immunizations and infectious diseases. Fischer MC, Editor in Chief. American Academy of Pediatrics, Elk Grove Village, IL, 2006.

Annual Epidemiological Report on Communicable Diseases in Europe. Report on the status of communicable diseases in the EU and EEA/EFTA countries. Amato-Gauci A, Ammon A, Editors. European Centre for Disease Prevention and Control, June 2007.

Offit PA, Bell LM. Vaccines: What you should know. 3rd Edition. John Wiley & Sons, Hoboken, NJ, 2003.

Smith MJ, Woods CR. On-time vaccine receipt in the first year does not adversely affect neuropsychological outcomes. Pediatrics 2010;125:1134–41.

Tozzi AE, Bisiacchi P, Tarantino V, et al. Neuropsychological performance 10 years after immunization in infancy with thimerosal-containing vaccines. Pediatrics 2009;123:475–82.

Chapter 10. Baby's on the Way:
Protect Your Unborn Baby with a Healthy Pregnancy

Grayson, ML. Infections in pregnant women. Medical Journal of Australia 2002; 176:229–36.

Harvey J, Dennis CL. Hygiene interventions for prevention of cytomegalovirus infection among childbearing women: Systematic review. Journal of Advanced Nursing 2008;63:440–50.

Klein JO, Remington JS. Current concepts of infections of the fetus and newborn infant. In: Infectious diseases of the fetus and newborn infant. Remington JS, Klein JO, Editors. 5th Edition. Saunders, Philadelphia, 2001.

Chapter 12. Supplements, Herbs, Organic Produce, and Probiotics:
Do They Protect You from Germs?

Consumer Reports. When it pays to buy organic. February 2006. Available at www.consumerreports.org/cro/food/diet-nutrition/organic-products.

Gardiner MD. Dietary supplement use in children: Concerns for efficacy and safety. American Family Physician 2005;71(6):1068–71.

Gardiner P, Kemper KJ. Herbs in pediatric and adolescent medicine. Pediatrics in Review 2000;21:44–57.

Goldin BR, Gorbach SL. Clinical indications for probiotics: An overview. Clinical Infectious Diseases 2008;46:S96–100.

Lara-Villoslada F, Olivares M, Sierra S, Rodriguez JM, Boza J, Xaus J. Beneficial effects of probiotic bacteria isolated from breast milk. British Journal of Nutrition 2007;98:S96–100.

Rex Gaskins H, Croix JA, Nakamura N, Nava GM. Impact of the intestinal microbiota on the development of mucosal defense. Clinical Infectious Diseases 2008;46:S80–86.

Saxelin M. Probiotic formulations and applications, the current probiotic market, and changes in the marketplace: A European perspective. Clinical Infectious Diseases 2008;46:S76–79.

Chapter 13. Wash Your Hands!
Personal and Household Hygiene for the Twenty-first Century

Gelfand EW. The hygiene hypothesis revisited: Pros and cons. Available at www .medscape.com/viewarticle/452170, accessed March 3, 2009.

International Scientific Forum on Home Hygiene. Guidelines for prevention of infection and cross infection in the domestic environment. 2nd Edition. Intramed Communications, Milan, Italy, 2004.

Kinnula S, Tapiainen T, Renko M, Uhari M. Safety of alcohol hand gel use among children and personnel at a child day care center. American Journal of Infection Control 2009;37:318–21.

Strachan DP. Hay fever, hygiene, and household size. British Medical Journal 1989; 299:1259–60.

Chapter 14. Myths and Truths: Does Science Back Up
Traditional Wisdom about Preventing Infections?

Pachter LM, Summer T, Fontan A, et al. Home-based therapies for the common cold among European American and ethnic minority families. Archives of Pediatric and Adolescent Medicine 1998;152:1083–88.

Rakover Y, Ben-Arye E, Goldstein LH. The treatment of respiratory ailments with essential oils of some aromatic medicinal plants. Harefuah (Abstract in English) 2008;147:783–88.

Sanu A, Eccles R. The effects of a hot drink on nasal airflow and symptoms of common cold and flu. Rhinology 2008;46:271–75.

Theis J, Koren G. Camphorated oil: Still endangering the lives of Canadian children. Canadian Medical Association Journal 1995;152:1821–24.

Uc A, Bishop WP, Sanders KD. Camphor hepatotoxicity. Southern Medical Journal 2000;93:596–98.

Zanker KS, Tolle W, Blumel G, Probst J. Evaluation of surfactant-like effects of commonly used remedies for colds. Respiration 1980;39:150–57.

Index

About the Author

Dr. Athena P. Kourtis is a pediatrician and a specialist in infectious diseases of children. She trained in Pediatrics and Pediatric Infectious Diseases at Hahnemann University, the Johns Hopkins University, and Emory University, in Immunology at the Pasteur Institute in Paris, and in Epidemiology and Public Health at the Johns Hopkins University. Dr. Kourtis currently holds academic appointments as an Associate Professor of Pediatrics at Emory University School of Medicine and at Eastern Virginia Medical School and is a scientist at the Centers for Disease Control and Prevention in Atlanta. She has practiced pediatrics and infectious disease medicine for fifteen years and has received many national and international awards and recognition for her research in pediatric immunology, infections, and HIV, including awards from the American Academy of Microbiology and the U.S. Federal Executive Board. She is a fellow of the American Academy of Pediatrics and the Infectious Diseases Society of America. Dr. Kourtis has published over one hundred original articles and book chapters, has edited medical books, and has led domestic and international clinical trials. Her experience as a pediatrician and also as a mother has given her the privilege of knowing first hand the most pressing questions and concerns of parents, and she can distill for parents the most important and accurate information they should know in order to protect their children's health. She lives in Atlanta with her husband and sons.